BREAST DISEASE
FOR
PRIMARY CARE
PHYSICIANS

BREAST DISEASE
FOR
PRIMARY CARE
PHYSICIANS

Bernard A. Eskin, MD
Allegheny University of the Health Sciences, Philadelphia, PA, USA

Sucha O. Asbell, MD
Albert Einstein Medical Center, Philadelphia, PA, USA

and
Lori Jardines, MD
Allegheny University of the Health Sciences, Philadelphia, PA, USA

The Parthenon Publishing Group
International Publishers in Medicine, Science & Technology

NEW YORK   LONDON

Library of Congress Cataloging-in-Publication Data
Breast disease for primary care physicians / By
Bernard A. Eskin, Sucha O. Asbell, and Lori
Jardines.
       p.   cm.
     Includes bibliographical references and index.
     ISBN 1-85070-744-8
     1. Breast—Diseases—Diagnosis. 2. Primary
care (Medicine).   3. Breast—Cancer—
Treatment. I. Eskin, Bernard A.   II. Asbell,
Sucha O.   III. Jardines, Lori.
    [DNLM: 1. Breast Diseases—diagnosis.
2. Breast Diseases—therapy. 3. Primary Health
Care—methods. WP 840 B82845 1998]
RG492.B74 1998
618.1′9—dc21
DNLM/DLC
for Library of Congress   98-22292
                         CIP

British Library Cataloguing in Publication Data
Breast disease for primary care physicians
  1. Breast – Diseases – Diagnosis 2. Breast –
  Diseases – Treatment
  I. Eskin, Bernard A. II. Asbell, Sucha O.
  III. Jardines, Lori
  618.1′9

ISBN 1-85070-744-8

Published in the USA by
The Parthenon Publishing Group Inc.
One Blue Hill Plaza
PO Box 1564, Pearl River
New York 10965, USA

Published in the UK and Europe by
The Parthenon Publishing Group Limited
Casterton Hall, Carnforth
Lancs., LA6 2LA, UK

Copyright © 1999 Parthenon Publishing Group

Printed by Butler & Tanner Ltd., Frome and
London, UK
Typeset by Martin Lister Publishing Services,
Carnforth, UK

Contents

List of Authors

Bernard A. Eskin, MD
Professor, Obstetrics/Gynecology and
  Reproductive Endocrinology/Infertility
Clinical Associate Professor, Psychiatry
Adjunct Professor, Pharmacology
Allegheny University of the Health Sciences
MCP-Hahnemann School of Medicine
3300 Henry Avenue
Philadelphia, PA 19129
USA

Sucha O. Asbell, MD
Professor, Department of Radiation Oncology
Temple University School of Medicine
Philadelphia, PA
and
Chairman, Department of Radiation Oncology
Albert Einstein Medical Center
5501 Old York Road
Philadelphia, PA 19141
USA

Lori Jardines, MD
Associate Professor, Department of Surgery
Chief, Division of Breast Surgery
Allegheny University of the Health Sciences
MCP Division
3300 Henry Avenue
Philadelphia, PA 19129
USA

List of Contributors

Barbara C. Cavanaugh, MD
Assistant Professor of Diagnostic Imaging
Temple University School of Medicine
Philadelphia, PA
and
Department of Radiology
Albert Einstein Medical Center
5501 Old York Road
Philadelphia, PA 19141
USA

Debra S. Copit, MD
Assistant Professor of Diagnostic Imaging
Temple University School of Medicine
Philadelphia, PA
and
Director, Gershon-Cohen Breast Center
Department of Radiology
Albert Einstein Medical Center
5501 Old York Road
Philadelphia, PA 19141
USA

Ierachmiel Daskal, MD
Chairman, Department of Pathology and
  Laboratory Medicine
Director, Clinical Pathology
Albert Einstein Medical Center
Philadelphia, PA 19141
USA

Pamela R. Edmonds, MD
Associate Professor of Pathology
Thomas Jefferson University Hospital
111 South 11th Street
Philadelphia, PA 19107
USA

Mark Granick, MD
Professor of Surgery
Chief, Division of Plastic Surgery
Allegheny University of the Health Sciences
MCP Division
3300 Henry Avenue
Philadelphia, PA 19129
USA

Preface

Several of our medical colleagues bemoan the fact that their participation in the care of their patients is limited because the diagnosis and treatment of breast diseases have become too complex. However, both for medical and legal considerations, they feel that care should be placed in the hands of specialists as soon as breast disease is diagnosed. At this crucial time the patient may consult her primary physician for information, advice and, often, solace. If the physician is familiar with the current status of each diagnosis and treatment these are more easily provided.

With this in mind, the present volume was conceived. We believe it provides the necessary information to help the reader in the assessment of the patient's condition and the resolution of conflicting ideas where over-abundant media coverage has confused the medical issues.

The senior authors consist of an obstetrician–gynecologist–endocrinologist, a radiation oncologist, and a breast surgeon. Despite this diversity of subspecialties, additional experts in other specific fields have been asked to contribute chapters. These are Cavanaugh (diagnostic imaging), Copit (interventional breast procedures), Edmonds (fine needle aspiration cytology), Daskal (pathology), and Granick (breast reconstruction).

We have followed the suggestions of several primary physicians who have tested our recommendations. We tried to include those problems and conditions most commonly seen in medical practice.

Writing this book has provided the authors with an opportunity to review and categorize most of the complexities of breast disease treatment. Nevertheless much remains to be learned and proven.

Bernard A. Eskin, MS, MD
Sucha O. Asbell, MD
Lori Jardines, MD
Philadelphia

Acknowledgements

The authors wish to thank the editors and staff of the Parthenon Publishing Group for their assistance, advice, and encouragement in this project. We are particularly grateful to the editor, Nat Russo, his associate, Roseann Caserio, and our scientific editor Dinah Alam, for their personal assistance in the presentation of our material. The difficult and frustrating job of sorting and collating the book was competently achieved by Lynn Eskin, to whom we give our heartfelt thanks.

B.A. Eskin
S.O. Asbell
L. Jardines

I personally would like to thank my wonderful husband, Lee Kaplan, for his patience and understanding in all of the late nights I had to keep to complete this project, and my incredible and very supportive secretary, Mitzi Ruggieri-Jones, who helped me to achieve and meet the deadlines.

L. Jardines

I personally thank my husband, Michael J. Asbell, for giving me the time and space to complete this effort. I also thank Lori Weinert and Nancy Bowes for their secretarial assistance.

S.O. Asbell

Anatomy of the breast

1

B.A. Eskin

Human mammary glands lie on the pectoralis muscles. They are essentially accommodated between the pectoralis muscle and the overlying skin, and encroach the area of the chest from the second rib to the sixth or seventh intercostal space. Laterally, they extend into the apical area and medially towards the lateral aspect of the sternum (Figure 1.1).

In the cross-section of the breast, it is noted that the skin superficially has two layers, with a thinned areola in the tissue center. The areolar region contains an elevated nipple, which has in its center apices through which the primary ducts open (Figure 1.2). Smooth muscle is arranged circularly and longitudinally below the areolar area, with potential for erection and contraction of the apices. There are usually 15–20 openings into the nipple, each representing a duct–lobule system. The nipple contains nerves, elastic tissue and muscle which activate the erectile patterns. The nipples hypertrophy and contract with nursing and sexual arousal. Around the circumference of the nipple–areolar complex, small glands secrete a thick lipid substance which protects the nursing mother from injury.

Below the skin, there is a thicker, fascial sheath which completely encases the underlying breast tissues from the skin to the pectoralis muscle fascia. The first layer below the fascia contains a good deal of fat, irregularly arranged as a protective coat through which the lactiferous (milk) ducts travel.

Within the breast, the smallest units are the internally located terminal ducts or acini, which initiate and produce the secretions. Acini are multicellular (two to four cell thicknesses) and myoepithelial structures which lie on the basement membranes. The myoepithelial cells seem similar to smooth muscle but are hormone-activated (Figure 1.3). Tertiary and secondary ducts (two-cell layered) extend from these terminal bud-like structures (acini) and eventually join to become the primary ducts which enter the areolar–nipple area. These tertiary, secondary, and primary ducts together with connective tissues and blood vessels form larger units called lobules. Each lobule has a primary duct termination.

The subdermal or superficial (primary) fat externally and the layer anterior to the pectoral muscle (secondary fat) essentially protect the active breast tissues. Genetic variability in size and form, often expressed by fat content and metabolism, exists. The superficial fat is based on hormonal and nutritional intake, while the secondary fat appears to be most affected by heredity.

During the ages of reproduction, ducts are firm, regular and easily distinguished. Surrounding the ducts are layers of elastic and fibrous tissues which permit the positioning of the ducts, and provide a mobile cushion.

EMBRYOLOGY

The breast is thought to originate as sweat gland tissue and as part of the integument. During the fifth fetal week (6–10 mm), the ectodermal primitive milk streaks appear on the embryo as a thickening on each side of the ventral midline, from the axilla to the groin. The primitive milk streaks regress (9–15 mm), usually remaining only in the region of the thorax, where they form a mammary ridge (Figure 1.4).

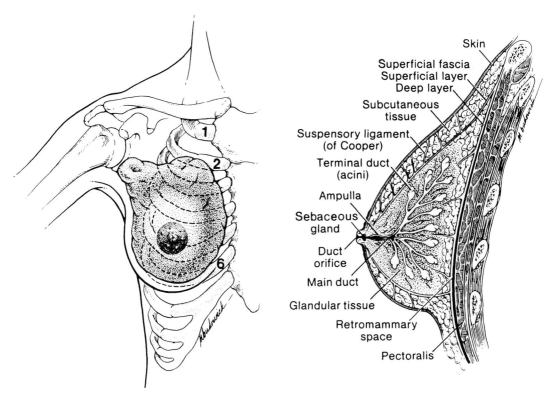

Figure 1.1 On the chest wall, the breast extends from the second to sixth ribs and from the lateral border of the sternum to the mid-axillary line. The long axis is toward the axilla, the tail of Spence. (From Egan RL. *Breast Imaging – Diagnosis and Morphology of Breast Diseases*. Philadelphia: W.B. Saunders Co., 1988, with permission)

Figure 1.2 Glandular and supporting framework of the breast.(From Egan RL. *Breast Imaging – Diagnosis and Morphology of Breast Diseases*. Philadelphia: W.B. Saunders Co., 1988, with permission)

Between the third and fourth month, bud-shaped primordia develop. At 16 weeks, desquamation of the epithelium results in the nipple groove. Further epithelial proliferations branch out into 15–25 bands and form the anlage of the ductal system and secretory alveoli. A secondary mammary anlage develops with the differentiation of hair follicle and sebaceous and sweat gland elements. Specialized apocrine glands also develop at this time to form Montgomery's glands surrounding the nipple.

Hormonally, the canalization stage requires sex hormones (secreted by the placenta) which enter the fetal circulation during weeks 20–32. Lobular alveolar structures contain colostrum in the third trimester. By term, 15–25 mammary ducts are formed. Capillaries develop into a complex vascular network within the connective tissue.

The lymphatic drainage of the breast is a significant and important factor in malignant disease. The lymph nodes are conventionally grouped in three layers, which are marked I, II, and III in Figure 1.5. Formerly, radical resection of the axillary nodes was an integral part of the classical radical mastectomy. This is seldom performed now, since it has not prolonged survival or time of first recurrence. Tumor-containing lymph nodes at level III are rarely present if those in levels I and II are negative. Most breast surgeons, therefore, resect only level I and II lymph nodes for staging purposes.

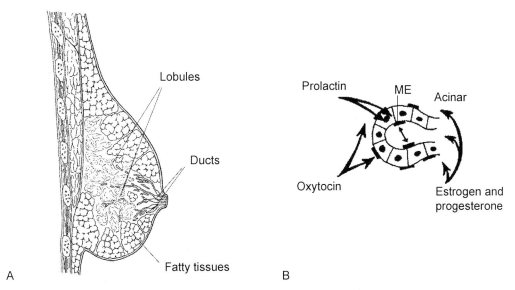

A

B

Figure 1.3 Secretory cells. The human breast. A, sagittal view; B, secretory cells in acinus; ME, myoepithelial cells. (From Eskin BA. Disorders of prolactin secretion. In *Issues in Reproductive Endocrinology*. Technical Newsletter of Becton Dickinson Immunodiagnostics, Orangeburg, NY, USA, 1984, with permission)

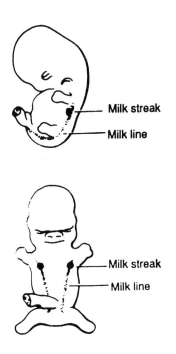

Figure 1.4 Milk streak development in the embryo. (From Wagner H. Topographische Anatomie der-weblichen Bust. In: Beller FK, ed. *Atlas der Mamma Chirurgie*. Stuttgart: Schattauer, 1985)

ABNORMAL BREAST DEVELOPMENT
Congenital abnormalities

The most frequently observed abnormality seen in both sexes is an accessory nipple (polythelia). Ectopic nipple tissue is often mistaken for a pigmented nevus, and may occur at any point along the embryonic milk streak (Figure 1.6) from the axilla to the groin. Rarely, true accessory mammary glands develop, which are most often located in the axilla (polymastia). During pregnancy and lactation, an accessory breast may swell; occasionally, if there is an associated nipple, it may function and cause diagnostic confusion.

A wide range of breast abnormalities have been described; however, most are not severe. *Hypoplasia* is the underdevelopment of the breast; congenital absence of a breast is termed *amastia*. When breast tissue is lacking but a nipple is present, the condition is termed *amazia*. *Amastia*, or marked breast hypoplasia, is associated with hypoplasia of the pectoral muscle in 90% of cases, although the reverse does not apply. Ninety-two per cent of women with pectoral muscle abnormalities have normal breasts.

3

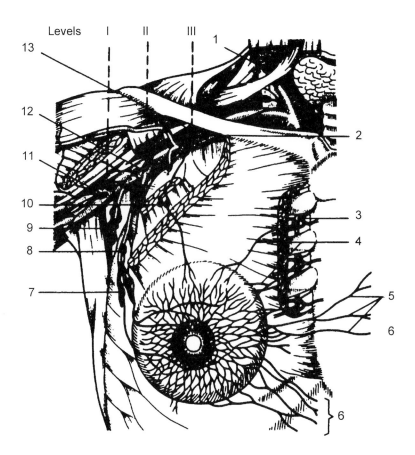

Figure 1.5 Lymph drainage of the breast. 1, Deep cervical nodes; 2, infraclavicular nodes; 3, sternal nodes; 4, pathway to the mediastinal nodes; 5, pathway to the contralateral breast; 6, pathway to the subdiaphragmatic nodes and liver; 7, anterior pectoral lymph nodes; 8, central axillary nodes; 9, subpectoral axillary nodes; 10, interpectoral nodes (Rotter's); 11, brachial vein nodes; 12, axillary vein nodes; 13, subclavian vein nodes. See text for definitions of lymph node levels I, II, and III. (From Mitchell GW, Bassett LW. *The Female Breast and its Disorders*. Baltimore: Williams and Wilkins, 1990, with permission)

Congenital abnormalities of the pectoral muscle are usually manifested by the lack of the lower third of the muscle and an associated deformity of the ipsilateral rib cage.

Acquired abnormalities

The most common cause of amazia is iatrogenic and avoidable. Injudicious biopsy during precocious breast development results in the excision of all or part of the breast bud, resulting in subsequent marked loss, deformity, and growth irregularities during puberty. The use of radiation therapy in prepubertal females to treat either intrathoracic disease or local hemangioma of the breast may also result in amazia. Traumatic injury of the developing breast, particularly severe cutaneous burns or similar damage, with subsequent contractures, may also result in abnormalities.

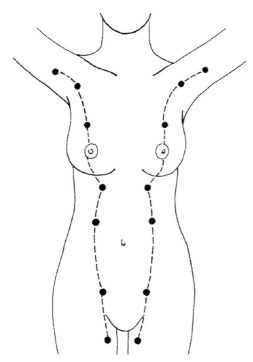

Figure 1.6 Representation of the embryonic milk lines showing sites where accessory breast tissue and supernumerary nipples arise

Table 1.1 Breast endocrinology

Substance	Development	Alveolar growth	Pubertal changes	Lactation
T3/T4	+	+	+	+
Iodine	+	+	+	+
Estrogen	–	–	+	+
Progesterone	–	–	+	+
Prolactin	–	–/+	+	+
Insulin	–	–	–	+
Cortisone	–	–	–	+

contractile elements for the expulsion of milk. The epithelial ducts and the myoepithelial component are the fastest proliferating tissues within the breast.

DEVELOPMENT OF THE FEMALE BREAST

The nipples and areolae are pigmented at birth. In the center of the breast plateau, the openings of 10–20 mammary ducts lead into large lactiferous sinuses, from which the primary branches gradually narrow towards the periphery. Colostral fluid, 'witch's milk', is produced in 80–90% of newborns, beginning on postpartum day 4–7, and may be expressed from the nipple. This secretion lasts for 3–4 weeks and is due to stimulation of the end vesicles by luteal and placental hormones, particularly estrogen and prolactin. Like mother's milk, repeated expression of colostrum can delay its cessation. After the first neonatal month, infant breast tissue regresses to approximately 4–8 mm in depth. No further growth occurs until puberty.

The mammary glands consist of four major tissues: fat, connective tissue, epithelium, and myoepithelial cells, which constitute the

NORMAL BREAST DEVELOPMENT DURING PUBERTY

Puberty in girls begins at the age of 10–12 years as a result of hypothalamic gonadotropin-releasing hormone (GnRH) secretion. The gonadotropic cells of the anterior pituitary respond to the pulsatile GnRH by secreting variable quantities of follicle-stimulating hormone (FSH) and luteinizing hormone (LH). FSH causes the primordial ovarian follicles to mature into graafian follicles, which secrete estrogens, mostly in the form of 17β-estradiol. All of these sex hormones are involved in inducing growth and maturation of the breasts and genital organs. It is apparent that many hormones are involved, and the four tissue types react differently to each (Table 1.1).

During the 18 months that follow menarche (the first vaginal bleeding), maturation of the primordial ovarian follicles occurs, but commonly does not result in ovulation. Ovarian estrogen synthesis and secretion continues, since no luteal phase occurs. The physiologic effect of estrogens on the maturing breast is through stimulation of longitudinal growth of ductal epithelium. The essential terminal ductules form buds which are the anlage of breast lobules. Simultaneously, periductal connective tissues increase in volume and elasticity, with

Table 1.2 Tanner stages of breast growth

Stage 1 The infantile stage, which persists from the immediate postnatal period until the onset of puberty.

Stage 2 The 'bud' stage. The breast and papilla are elevated as a small mound, and the diameter of the areola is increased. This appearance is the first indication of pubertal development on the breast.

Stage 3 The breast and areola are further enlarged and present an appearance similar to that of a small adult mammary gland, with a continuous rounded contour.

Stage 4 The areola and papilla continue to expand and form a secondary mound projecting above the corpus of the breast.

Stage 5 The typical adult stage with a smooth rounded contour, the secondary mound present in Stage 4 having disappeared.

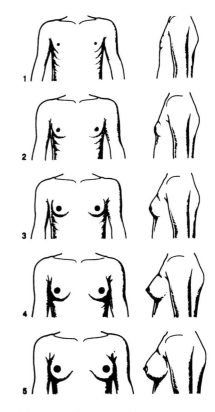

Figure 1.7 Tanner's stages of breast development

enhanced vascularity and fat deposition. These changes, induced by this hyperestrinism, result from ovarian follicles remaining immature and anovulatory. By 18 months after menarche, follicles will mature and ovulate with corpus luteum formation (luteal phase) releasing progesterone. While estrogen alone induces a pronounced ductular growth, progesterone requires estrogen presence for its receptor action. These two hormones together produce the full ductular–lobular–alveolar development characteristic of active mammary tissues.

There are marked individual variations in the development and maturation of the breast. These are guided by genetic and receptor responses, making it difficult critically to categorize histologic changes only on the basis of age. For this reason, clinical breast development by age has been characterized by external morphologic changes. The classical phases for breast development described by Tanner as five stages of growth are used by most clinicians (Table 1.2 and Figure 1.7).

In recent epidemiological studies in several countries, differences in age for menarche and end of breast development were noted. In the United States (1996), the median age of menarche was 12.5 years and the end of breast development was 14.2 years. In Tanner's study, the median age of menarche was 13.5, and the end point of breast development was later. The difference in the age of menarche was not statistically significant. Thelarche (onset of breast growth) was the first sex characteristic to appear, followed by pubarche (genital hair), axillarche (axillary hair), and finally menarche.

The breast is a skin appendage contained within layers of superficial fascia. In Western females, breast differentiation ceases 2 years after menarche, since by that time, duct, lobules, and alveoli have been defined. The size, form, and consistency of the breast are determined not only by these major parts but also by connective and adipose tissue. Each of these elements can be predominant in a given individual.

Fat deposits are primarily responsible for breast shape. The well-formed breasts in individuals with testicular feminization predominantly contain adipose tissue. The fat loss in menopause may be modified by estrogen therapies.

MICROSCOPIC ANATOMY OF THE MATURING AND ADULT BREAST

In the immature breast, the ducts and alveoli are lined by two layers of epithelium which consist of (1) a basal cuboidal layer and (2) a flattened surface layer. After estrogens become active at puberty and thereafter, the epithelial layers proliferate, becoming multilayered. Three alveolar cell types have been classified: superficial (luminal) A cells, basal B cells (chief cells), and myoepithelial cells.

Superficial A cells are dark, basophilic-staining cells that are rich in ribosomes. Superficial cells undergo intercellular dehiscence, with swelling of the mitochondria, and become groups, forming buds within the lumen. Basal B cells are the major cell type in mammary epithelium. They are clear, with an ovoid nucleus without nucleoli. Where the basal cells are in contact with the lumen, there are microvilli on the cell membrane. Intracytoplasmic filaments are similar to those in myoepithelial cells, suggesting their differentiation toward that cell type. Growth may, therefore, be in a peripheral direction from the lumen.

Myoepithelial cells are located around alveoli and small excretory milk ducts between the inner aspect of the basement membrane and the tunica propria. Myoepithelial cells (Figure 1.3) are arranged in a branching, starlike fashion. The sarcoplasm contains filaments 50–80 μm in diameter; these myofilaments are inserted by hemidesmosomes into the basal membrane. These cells are not activated by nerves but are stimulated by the non-steroidal hormones, prolactin and oxytocin. The normal and pathologic microscopic changes in the breast are further described and illustrated in Chapter 12.

Bibliography

Birkenfeld A, Kase NG. Functional anatomy and physiology of the female breast (review). *Obstet Gynecol Clin N Am* 1994;21:433–44

Egan RL. *Breast Imaging – Diagnosis and Morphology of Breast Diseases*. Philadelphia: W.B. Saunders, 1988

Eskin BA. Disorders of prolactin secretion. In *Issues in Reproductive Endocrinology*. RIA, 1984

Eskin BA. *The Menopause: Comprehensive Management*, 3rd edn. New York: McGraw Hill, 1995: 211–28

Healy W, Hodge W. *Surgical Anatomy*. Philadelphia: B.C. Decker, 1990:41–52

Logan-Young W, Hoffman NY. *Breast Cancer: A Practical Guide to Diagnosis, Volume 1: Procedures*. Rochester, NY: Mt. Hope Publishing Company, 1994: 15–30

Mitchell GW, Bassett LW. *The Female Breast and its Disorders*. Baltimore: Williams and Wilkins, 1990: 1–12

Spratt JS, Tobin GR. Gross anatomy of the breast. In Donegan WL, Spratt JS, eds. *Cancer of the Breast*. Philadelphia: W.B. Saunders, 1994:22–42

Vorherr H. *The Breast*. New York: Academic Press, 1974

Wagner H. Topographische Anatomie der weblichen Bust. In Beller FK, ed. *Atlas der Mamma Cirurgie*. Stuttgart: Schattauer, 1985

Williams PL, Warwick R, Dyson M, *et al*, eds. *Gray's Anatomy*, 37th edn. New York: Churchill Livingstone, 1993:1129–36

Endocrinology of the breast 2

B.A. Eskin

INTRODUCTION

The breast is a major target organ for the reproductive hormones. Throughout the body, estrogen and progesterone stimulate intracellular responses. These same hormones have specific effects on growth and metabolism in the ducts and connective tissues of the breast. Other hormones have secondary effects on the mammary functions that are fundamental to reproduction. However, regardless of these practical aspects, the breast continues to command much attention because of emotional and sexual responses generated by hormones.

THE BREAST AS AN ENDOCRINE ORGAN

Mammary glands are unique endocrine organs that undergo growth, differentiation, and lactation in response to hormones. The hormonal regulation of mammogenesis occurs throughout fetal, adolescent, and adult life. The endocrine milieu of pregnancy has an important effect on the breast that is critical for normal lactation. After delivery of the newborn, a complex neuroendocrine feedback system controls milk ejection and maintains lactation until weaning. Involution follows, with a gradual return to the resting state, until pregnancy again stimulates a cycle of secretory activity.

Biologically, the overall major function of the human breast is the preparation and delivery of milk, resulting in the ability to feed one's young. The breast has the capacity through biochemical intracellular units to synthesize milk, a highly nutritious substance for the newborn.

Milk is delivered to the baby through a duct system which runs through the breast and terminates in large sinuses externally at the nipple. These purely independent activities require internal and external stimuli.

Ducts run singly throughout the tissues of the breast, beginning internally with the terminal duct or acinar which contains the responsible synthetic plant. These active tissues comprise 20% of the breast and are essentially elastic, pliable and relatively soft. The remainder of the breast consists of layers of adipose and connective tissue components which are firmer and have a function to protect and support. Any of these components may age, atrophy, become diseased or abnormal. These processes may bring about benign and malignant changes which can lead to pain, illness and death. Breasts are anatomically part of the integument and thus can be readily examined for clinical abnormalities. In the reproductive years, mammary gland tissues are functional, with characteristic cycles which result in an increased tendency for temporal symptoms accompanied by tissue changes. When reproduction wanes, the breast irregularities that occur are more likely to be serious, and malignancies increase.

GENERAL BREAST ENDOCRINOLOGY

In the pre-pubertal girl, a primordial cyst develops by the fourth to sixth year, and by the eighth year, when ovarian estrogen first begins to be secreted (thelarche), the differentiation of primary and secondary ducts becomes visible.

Growth and development of the breast is affected by many substances. The most important ones include thyroid hormone, iodine, insulin, cortisol and eventually reproductive steroids, estrogen and progesterone (Table 1.1). By menarche, breast tissues are close to full maturity and may be assessed according to size, appearance and nipple growth as shown in the Tanner phases (Chapter 1). Tertiary ducts, though rudimentary at first, should be present; they have the capability of milk synthesis. Throughout the reproductive years when estrogen and progesterone cyclicity occurs, the lining cells of the ducts react to these hormones resulting in hypertrophy and hyperplasia. Specifically, estrogen increases the duct size by hypertrophy of the lining cells, while progesterone causes hyperplasia of these cells by increasing chemical activity of prelactation compounds within the terminal ducts.

As estrogen reaches its apex near mid-cycle, a third hormone, prolactin, is secreted from the pituitary, the level of which increases and remains elevated until estrogen decreases. Prolactin has the ability to bind lactalbumin to casein in the terminal ducts, which results in the synthesis of milk.

During a non-pregnant cycle, the amount of ductile secretions generated is minimal and they are usually absorbed through the duct lining. Periodic evidence of inspissated milk on the nipple follows this pattern. If the secretion does not flow out, it may be impeded within the duct, which results in a fluid-filled segment. Ductal damage which may then occur leads to acute or chronic fibrocystic areas because of the resulting formation of a fibrous protective tissue about the traumatized area. When these ductal changes occur, the patient may become uncomfortable and this discomfort continues until estrogen decreases. Progesterone increases the duct size in association with estrogen, which in most cases increases the pain during the premenstrual period.

During the latter half of pregnancy and postpartum, prolactin gradually increases exponentially, resulting in greater potential synthesis and availability of milk (Figure 2.1). However, the high levels of estrogen from the placenta during pregnancy prevent abundant milk secretion during the latter months of gestation. The flow of milk postpartum is maintained by newborn sucking, stimulating the sensory pathways from the nipple to the brain. Posterior pituitary secretions of oxytocin and possibly vasopressin are the intermediate hormones. These act on the myoepithelial cells surrounding the terminal ducts and cause initiation of milk flow (Figure 1.3).

HORMONAL DEVELOPMENT OF THE HUMAN BREAST – MAMMOGENESIS

Many hormones are involved in mammary development, which begins in the early fetus. These include prolactin, growth hormones, thyroid-stimulating hormone (TSH), luteinizing hormone (LH), human placental lactogen (hPL), ovarian and adrenal steroids, and insulin. While specific hormonal requirements are unknown, administration of minimal estrogen induces breast development in the human at any phase of life. Clinically, repetitive suckling stimuli induce lactation in nulliparous females in the absence of pregnancy or exogenous hormone supplementation, and this technique may be used for nursing in adoptions or genetic mothers in surrogate pregnancies.

Embryonic and prepubertal development

The breast is identified 6 weeks after conception as an ectodermal thickening along the ventrolateral aspect of the fetus. With cell growth, a mammary ridge is formed which soon differentiates into localized areas representing paired glands. The major pair of glands develops in the thoracic (pectoral) region, but supernumerary nipples with breast tissues may develop anywhere along the 'milk' ridge (Figure 1.4).

Epithelial cell proliferation and penetration into the underlying mesenchyme form the clinically important, but primitive, mammary bud. During the second trimester, projections of

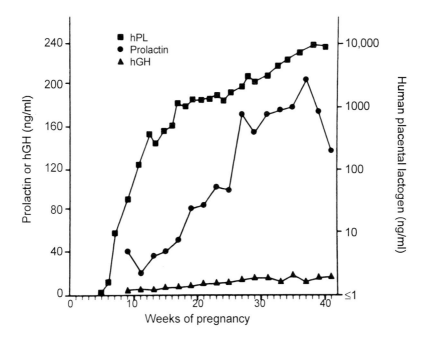

Figure 2.1 Mean values of plasma prolactin, human growth hormone (hGH), and human placental lactogen (hPL) during normal pregnancy. (From Kaplan CR. Endocrinology of the breast. In *The Female Breast and its Disorders*. Baltimore: Williams and Wilkins, 1990, 24 with permission)

ectoderm form the primary sprouts (15–25 in humans), which will eventually elongate and arborize to form the lactiferous ducts. This initial growth is independent of maternal or fetal hormones.

Lactiferous ducts canalize late in fetal life and form two layers of epithelial cells: an inner layer of cells which is secretory and an outer layer of cells that results in the myoepithelium. The main lactiferous ducts are present in the fetus. Influenced by fetal prolactin and placental steroids, limited ductal differentiation and secretory activity occur in late gestation (Figure 2.1).

There are no histologic or functional differences between the human male and female breast until puberty. At birth, all newborns may show breast secretions ('witch's milk') for several days. After birth, the epithelial cells revert to an undifferentiated state and remain quiescent until puberty. Little ductal growth is seen during childhood, with no lobuloalveolar development at all.

Puberty

Estrogen levels rise prior to menarche, usually around 8 years of age, when thelarche accompanies lactiferous duct proliferation. Breast development occurs due to deposition of periglandular adipose tissue with concurrent formation by the stromal connective tissue of the interlobular septa. Estrogen appears to be necessary for mammary development in women, as breast enlargement fails to occur in girls with gonadal dysgenesis at the age of puberty. Estrogen stimulates ductal proliferation but not lobuloalveolar development, the latter also being dependent on progesterone presence.

When regular ovulatory cycles begin, estrogen and progesterone levels rise, which results in increased blood flow and interlobular edema. A moderate degree of ductal and lobular proliferation vacillates with each follicular and luteal phase. As described in later chapters, this cyclic phenomenon is responsible for the benign and

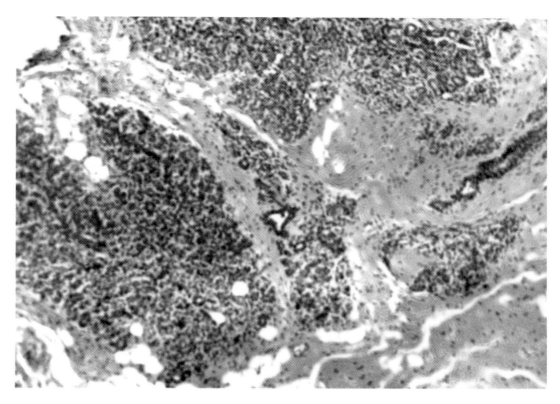

Figure 2.2 Photomicrograph of female breast tissues (×6.8). Perimenopausal breast section showing active duct and stromal areas (age 32 years). (Courtesy of C. Grotkowski and W. Battisti)

malignant changes. Just prior to menses, concurrent milk discharge or an evaporated residue on the nipple may occur. A reduction in the number and size of glandular cells occurs with menstruation. At this time there is a loss of edema, a minimal decrease in breast size, and diminished palpable duct irregularities, an ideal time for examination of the breast and the chest wall.

During early adulthood, similar endocrine changes are encountered. There is evidence of hormonal intensity as the average estrogen levels appear to increase until the middle of the third decade. This action is responsible for the regular cycles encountered as well as the enlarging breast contour. The latter is caused by the greater growth of the anterior fat deposits in response to increasing hormone levels. Pregnancy modifications, described later in this chapter, follow the same sequences from shortly after puberty until menopause, with little variation.

PREGNANCY

The breasts become most active in preparation for lactation. Early in the first trimester, mammary epithelial cells proliferate, and ductal hypertrophy and branching are initiated. The ducts invade the fat pads, and the ductal end buds differentiate. Maturing mammary glands occur in clusters of epithelial cells (lobules) organized into a sphere (alveolus). This growth is accompanied by increased mammary blood flow, interstitial water, and electrolyte concentrations. The proliferation seen in the lobuloalveolar structures occurs throughout pregnancy.

During the second trimester, the cells become single-layered and the lumina begin to dilate in the alveoli. Lymphocytes, plasma cells, and eosinophils collect in the interstitial spaces. Increased vascular luminal diameters and formation of new capillaries around the mammary lobules result in an enhanced mammary blood supply.

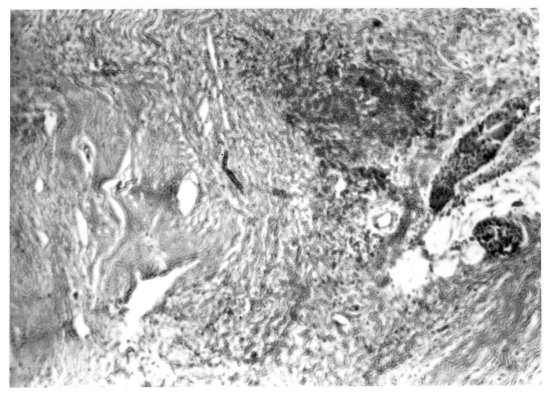

Figure 2.3 Photomicrograph of female breast tissues (×6.8). Menopausal breast section with atrophic and inactive tissues (age 69 years). (Courtesy of C. Grotkowski and W. Battisti)

During the last trimester, the ductal secretory cells fill with fat droplets, and the alveoli distend and begin synthesizing a proteinaceous, eosinophilic secretion – colostrum. Epithelial proliferation of the breasts plateaus as the alveolar epithelium prepares for its secretory function.

Hormonal control of mammary development during pregnancy

Several hormones increase markedly during pregnancy and significantly affect mammary development. 17β-Estradiol (E_2) is an essential hormone which is required for mammary growth and epithelial proliferation, particularly during pregnancy (Table 1.1). E_2 stimulates prolactin release and increases the number of breast prolactin receptors (Figure 2.1).

During pregnancy, progesterone stimulates lobuloalveolar growth (hyperplasia) while sup-pressing secretory activity. High progesterone levels inhibit lactose synthetase and milk protein (casein) mRNA synthesis *in vitro*. Progesterone plays a positive role in differentiation by sensitizing mammary cells to the effects of insulin and growth factors, and prepares the mammary glands for lactogenesis.

A confusing aspect of breast endocrinology during pregnancy has been the relationship of human prolactin to human placental lactogen (hPL). Maternal prolactin and placental hPL increase concurrently during pregnancy and reach peak levels prior to parturition (Figure 2.1). Human prolactin and hPL have considerable amino acid similarities (13%), and the lactogenic activity of the two hormones is alike, since either hormone is sufficient for providing breast growth and development in humans. The amino acid sequence of hPL resembles human growth hormone (hGH).

Several hormones are not essential for ductal or alveolar growth, but are actively enhanced during pregnancy. Glucocorticoid levels increase during pregnancy, primarily due to a decreased clearance rate, an increase in corticosteroid-binding globulin, and an increase in unbound steroids. Glucocorticoids enhance formation of lobules during pregnancy. Insulin acts in synergy with prolactin to stimulate terminal differentiation of insulin-sensitive mammary cells *in vitro*, and in high concentrations insulin acts as a mitogen.

Thyroid hormone and iodine, while not necessary for ductal growth, are essential for alveolar growth. During pregnancy iodine increases in the breast tissues, particularly through the second and third trimesters. Iodine metabolism seems to parallel the prolactin surges. Thyroid hormones increase the responsiveness of mammary cells to prolactin and may improve lactational performance. Iodine is directly involved in milk secretions, and is vital to fetal growth and development.

Hormonal effects on postpartum lactogenesis

Lactogenesis is evident prepartum and at delivery. During the second trimester, enzymatic and cytologic differentiation of the mammary epithelium and limited milk secretion begin. First, the concentration of enzymes and other substrates, specific for milk secretion, increase within the alveolar cells. Secondarily, lactose, casein, α-lactalbumin and lactose synthetase are produced by mammary epithelial cells. Thereafter secretions are seen in the alveolar lumen, and the breast becomes engorged.

During delivery, progesterone and hPL levels fall, but estrogen, prolactin, prostaglandin $F_{2\alpha}$, oxytocin, and glucocorticoids, thyroxine and iodine levels increase. These rising hormone levels do not initiate lactation, since even though prolactin levels peak shortly before delivery, lactation does not occur. Estrogen inhibits puerperal lactation by inhibiting prolactin receptor activity, which prevents any

secretory activity of the alveolar epithelium from occurring. The removal of the placenta at parturition causes estrogen secretion to cease and, therefore, within a day, the barrier for lactogenic hormone action on milk synthesis is removed. Progesterone withdrawal is the most likely lactogenic trigger mechanism when prolactin becomes biologically available. Recent studies have shown that prolactin and glucocorticoids are bound to similar receptors on the lining epithelial cells, and promote lactogenic activity.

During the first few postpartum days after placental steroids have disappeared from the maternal serum, variable quantities of colostrum are secreted. Gradually, this converts to mature milk, and copious milk secretion starts on the third or fourth postpartum day. A neurogenic signal is required to maintain lactation, and is provided by periodic infant or mechanical sucking. After 12 weeks breast milk synthesis declines to a threshold level, despite appropriate hormonal and milk suckling activity.

DISORDERS OF LACTATION

Normal prolactin activity

As described above, prolactin is essential for the initiation of lactation. Prolactin levels increase steadily throughout gestation, reaching an average of 200–300 ng/ml at term (Figure 2.1). However, lactogenesis does not occur early in human gestation because of the described inhibitory effects of estrogen and probably progesterone on prolactin receptors in the epithelial cells of the alveoli. The effect of prolactin on these mammary cells is mediated through specific hormone-binding receptors, whose numbers remain relatively constant throughout pregnancy, affected only by estrogen levels. Since prolactin, like estrogen, increases the concentration of its own receptor, a predelivery surge of prolactin is required if lactogenesis is to occur.

In postpartum women who breastfeed, the basal prolactin levels remain elevated for 1–2 weeks and may exhibit further smaller increases shortly after suckling. When not breastfeeding, prolactin levels fall rapidly, declining to pre-pregnancy levels within 4–6 weeks. Breastfeeding causes the basal prolactin level to remain elevated from 2 weeks to 3 months postpartum. After the third postpartum month, these levels become normal as well, and only small increases occur with suckling. The median prolactin levels depend on frequency and duration of suckling, especially in long-term nursing. When breastfeeding provides the majority of nutrition for the infant, the basal prolactin levels may vary greatly. Administration of bromocriptine (a dopamine agonist) to women at any time postpartum will decrease circulating prolactin levels and completely inhibit lactation.

Prolactin is thus shown to be required for initiation and maintenance of lactation.

Lactation failure

Lactation failure most often results from inadequate sucking by the infant and/or feedings that are too infrequent or of too short duration to stimulate milk supply. The introduction of supplemental food further jeopardizes the tenuous supply–demand control of milk synthesis, and milk availability declines further. Proper education and support with appropriate intervention usually prevents this decline in milk yields and ensures adequate lactation in the majority of motivated mothers.

Anatomical or pathological medical barriers to lactation are rare (see Chapter 1). Prompt identification of the abnormality is important to prevent malnutrition in a breastfed infant. While augmentation mammoplasty rarely interferes with successful lactation, reduction mammoplasty prevents normal milk drainage. The latter involves unavoidable autotransplantation of the nipple, disrupting the innervation of both the nipple and areola with severance of the lactiferous ducts as they enter the nipple.

Lactational insufficiency due to inadequate mammary glandular tissue has been described by several authors.

Galactorrhea

Galactorrhea is defined as the secretion of milk under non-physiologic circumstances. The amount of milk secreted varies greatly, and can be either spontaneous or more commonly a result of manual expression. Diagnostically, galactorrhea occurs alone or in association with amenorrhea, ovulatory dysfunction, and infertility. Non-puerperal galactorrhea has been associated with a variety of endocrine and non-endocrine disorders (Table 2.1).

Galactorrhea is usually diagnosed as a breast response to increased serum prolactin levels. Occasionally, hyperresponsiveness to normal prolactin levels has been seen. The primary diagnostic problem with an elevated serum prolactin is identifying pituitary-secreting adenomas. The availability of computerized tomography (CT) scans and magnetic resonance imaging (MRI) has made accurate diagnoses easier, although false-positive findings may be reported. Diagnosis is confounded by a wide variety of drugs and organic disorders that are associated with hyperprolactinemia (see Table 2.2).

Treatment of galactorrhea

Patients with galactorrhea, in the absence of menstrual dysfunction or hyperprolactinemia, may be followed with reassurance with yearly prolactin determinations. If galactorrhea is severe or if fertility is the prime goal, reduction of prolactin with bromocriptine or other dopamine agonists is the treatment of choice.

An elevated serum prolactin level without a demonstrable pituitary tumor, central nervous system disease, or other recognized causes of increased prolactin secretion has been described as idiopathic. A normal sella turcica CT scan excludes the presence of a microadenoma, although very small (<1 mm) adenomas may be missed. Long-term follow-up of patients with idiopathic hyperprolactinemia has confirmed that eventual tumor development is unlikely.

Table 2.1 Pathologic causes of inappropriate prolactin secretion

Structural hypothalamic lesions
    Craniopharyngioma
    Sarcoidosis
    Irradiation
    Head trauma
    Metastatic or primary neoplasms
    Surgical stalk section
Functional hypothalamic–pituitary disorders
Structural pituitary lesions
    Prolactinomas
    Empty-sella syndrome
    Acromegaly
    Cushing's disease
Endocrine–metabolic disorders
    Hypothyroidism, primary
    Addison's disease
    Adrenal carcinoma or hyperplasia
    Renal disease
    Nelson's syndrome
    Sheehan's syndrome
Chest wall trauma or infection
Other described causes
    Hysterectomy/oophorectomy
    Dilatation/curettage
    Polycystic ovarian syndrome
    Pseudotumor cerebri
    Pseudocyesis
Ectopic production
    Bronchogenic carcinoma
    Hypernephroma

Table 2.2 Pharmacologic causes of inappropriate prolactin secretion

Estrogens/progestogens
Dopamine receptor blockers
    Phenothiazines
    Haloperidol
    Metoclopramide
    Sulpiride
    Domperidone
    Methadone
Dopamine reuptake inhibitors
    Amphetamine
    Tricyclic antidepressants
Dopamine receptor stimulants
    Apomorphine
Dopamine-depleting agents
    Reserpine
    Alpha-methyldopa
    Monoamine oxidase inhibitors
Histamine H_2-receptor antagonists
    Cimetidine

The goals of therapy for prolactin-secreting tumors include a reduction in tumor mass, preservation of normal pituitary function, restoration of fertility in anovulatory women, and elimination of troublesome lactation. Modes of therapy include irradiation, surgery, drug therapy, and close periodic observation.

MENOPAUSE

With menopause, almost all of the tissues of the breast show the marked effects of the absence of estrogen and/or progesterone. Changes attributable to the loss of reproductive steroid hormones as opposed to those which are secondary to aging can be readily identified. The breast response may separate the effects of these two events in the mature years.

Breast anatomy becomes architecturally disturbed with the onset of the menopause. This results in a number of unpredictable tissue changes when replacement hormones are used. While benign histologically, the tissues lose the characteristics of the reproductive breast and often the modifications become difficult to diagnose with the usual non-invasive techniques (Figure 2.2).

Estrogen secretions decrease minimally from the age of approximately 28 years, moderately after 36, and acutely after the age of 42 years. Both estrogen and progesterone receptor systems are reduced when estrogen is lacking. Breast tissues show an initial loss of subcutaneous fat and connective tissues, while the duct system becomes inactive and eventually degenerates. This starts with a thinning of the cellular linings, particularly in the secondary and tertiary ducts. The fibrous tissue and elastic tissues eventually disintegrate and do so in a manner which often appears dysfunctional (Figure 2.2). The skin may become thin with dryness and wrinkling due to the aging process. These changes are non-hormonal and are brought about primarily by cellular degeneration with an inability to re-establish itself. The nipple loses some of its vascularity, and thus changes from a red appearance to a light pink.

The elastic tissues are fully responsible for breast support and a reduction is the cause of the reduced firmness which leads to complaints of sagging breasts. There is minimal muscular tissue initially and this is reduced or lost by the time of the climacteric. Obese patients have an increase in systemic estrone from available extra-ovarian androgen metabolism. Estrone, while a relatively weak estrogen, sometimes retains a semi-active state in the breasts for a long period of time after menopause. The prepectoral fat tissues remain for at least 10 years following menopause, while superficial fat layers dissipate almost immediately because of the loss of estrogen. This results in a caved-in and elongated appearance of the breast which is usually partially reversed with estrogen replacement therapy.

Postmenopausal hormone replacement therapy (HRT) and breast cancer

Postmenopausal hormone replacement has many significant benefits. Side-effects and contraindications to the hormones eliminate only a small percentage of women for whom this therapy would be useful. However, the risk of breast cancer serves as a serious deterrent for both initiating and continuing HRT for a large population.

Unfortunately, there are no definitive data available concerning this important medical issue in any prospective randomized study to date. Several useful summaries have been prepared which provide epidemiological correlations with large select groups. In order to advise a patient concerning menopausal hormonal therapy, a full evaluation of her personal genetic and health history is necessary.

Generally, estrogen is not given to patients with breast cancer, which reflects elevated estrogen receptor numbers and activity. Treatment with anti-estrogens is usually employed for limited periods and often bilateral ovariectomy is recommended to reduce intrinsic estrogen. Additionally, the use of progesterone is effective only for protection against endometrial cancer and seems neutral concerning breast malignancy.

An important clinical research project, the Woman's Health Initiative, is underway. Until further information is available, clinical judgement should be used to assess the trade-offs between risks and benefits.

Bibliography

Colditz GA, Hankinson SR, Hunter DJ, *et al.* The use of estrogens and progestins and the risk of breast cancer in postmenopausal women. *N Engl J Med* 1995;332:1589–93

Collaborative Group on Hormonal Factors in Breast Cancer. Breast cancer and hormonal contraceptives: collaborative reanalysis of individual data on 53 297 women with breast cancer and 100 239 women without breast cancer from 54 epidemiological studies. *Lancet* 1996;347:1713

Dreicer R, Wilding G. Steroid hormone agonists and antagonists in the treatment of cancer. *Cancer Invest* 1992;10:27

Forsyth IA. The mammary gland (review). *Baillière's Clin Endocrinol Metab* 1991;5:809–32

Fowler PA, Casey CG, Cameron GG. Cyclic changes in composition and volume of the breast during the menstrual cycle, measured by magnetic resonance imaging. *Br J Gynaecol* 1991;97:595–602

Kaplan CR. Endocrinology of the breast. In *The Female Breast and its Disorders*. Baltimore: Williams and Wilkins, 1990; 24

Laya MB, Larson EB, Taplin SH, *et al.* Effect of estrogen replacement therapy on the specificity and sensitivity of screening mammography. *J Natl Cancer Inst* 1996;88:643

Newcomb PA, Longnecker MP, Storer BE, *et al.* Long-term hormone replacement therapy and risk of breast cancer in postmenopausal women. *Am J Epidemiol* 1995;142:788–95

Simpson HW, Griffiths K, McArdle C. The luteal heat cycle of the breast in health. *Breast Cancer Res Treatment* 1993;27:239–45

von Schoultz B, Soderqvist G, Tani E, *et al.* Effects of female sex steroids on breast tissue. *Eur J Obstet Gynecol Reprod Biol* 1993;49:55

Breast pain

3

L. Jardines

Breast pain, also known as mastodynia or mastalgia, is a very common condition which affects many women at some point during their lives. In most patients, however, it is relatively short-lived, is not severe and does not require medical attention. Breast pain is divided into three subgroups: cyclical, non-cyclical and chest wall pain. Of patients seen in one mastalgia clinic, 85% were felt to have mild mastalgia and 15% had severe mastalgia. Within the group with severe mastalgia, 80% was cyclical, 10% was non-cyclical and 10% was secondary to chest wall pain. In one series, 21% of the women surveyed rated their breast pain as severe and less than half sought medical attention. The reason for patients not seeking medical advice for this problem is unclear and may be related to attitudes of medical professionals towards patients with this complaint.

CATEGORIES OF MASTALGIA

Cyclical mastalgia accounts for 67–80% of cases of breast pain. It is generally bilateral and described as dull, achy or burning. It is less commonly described as being unilateral. The pain is most often greatest in the upper outer quadrants of the breasts and may be referred to the medial aspect of the upper arm. Most women will give a history of bilateral mastalgia which begins 7–10 days premenstrually and resolves with menses. In the severe situation, the patient will have only a few days to 2 weeks during the course of the month which are pain-free. It most commonly occurs during the third and fourth decades of life and resolves spontaneously in approximately 22% of patients. In

nearly half of the patients it resolves with menopause. Women with cyclical mastalgia who require drug treatment generally respond to hormonal therapy. For these reasons, it has been proposed that there is a hormonal basis for cyclical mastalgia, although the pathogenesis for the process is not understood.

Non-cyclical mastalgia accounts for 10–26% of cases of breast pain. It occurs in both pre- and postmenopausal women and is unrelated to the menstrual cycle, with a peak incidence of approximately 10 years greater than patients with cyclical mastalgia. The discomfort is often described as a burning sensation which is generally retroareolar or in the upper outer quadrant and is unilateral. Non-cyclical mastalgia resolves spontaneously in 50% of patients. The success rate in treating non-cyclical mastalgia is significantly less than that seen with cyclical breast pain.

Chest wall discomfort is generally manifested by pain at the costochondral junction or along the ribs, and accounts for 7–10% of patients presenting with breast pain. It is important to distinguish true breast pain from pain associated with the musculoskeletal system, since the evaluation and treatment will be different.

EVALUATION OF MASTALGIA

A thorough history should be performed to determine the location and extent, as well as the timing, of the breast pain during the course of the menstrual cycle. A dietary history should be elicited and a careful drug history should be obtained. During the course of the history, it is necessary to try to distinguish cyclical from non-cyclical mastalgia. The patient should also receive a careful clinical breast examination. If a discrete mass is identified, it should be evaluated by breast imaging studies (mammography and/or ultrasonography, depending upon the patient's age). If it is a cyst, it can be easily aspirated and if it is solid, fine needle aspiration for cytology should be performed. In the majority of patients, there will be no suspicious findings on clinical examination and on mammography.

Pain is not a common presenting complaint in women with breast cancer and it is the only presenting complaint in 2.3–7% of patients who are diagnosed with this disease. Breast pain secondary to an underlying breast malignancy is generally unilateral, localized to a specific point, and persistent. Patients with mild mastalgia who have a negative breast examination and mammogram require only reassurance that there is no evidence of malignancy, and no additional intervention is necessary. For those patients with severe mastalgia and no evidence of malignancy on initial screening, it is useful to provide a pain chart which allows them to document the level of pain they experience on a daily basis and record the date of the onset of menses for two consecutive menstrual cycles. This will allow the pain to be categorized into either cyclical or non-cyclical. Women with unilateral or non-cyclical mastalgia should be referred to a breast specialist.

ETIOLOGY OF MASTALGIA

There have been no specific histologic findings after a breast biopsy which can be associated with an increased incidence of breast pain. Other etiologies which have been suggested are dietary and hormonal factors. It had been reported that consumption of methylxanthines, caffeine, theophylline and theobromine, was associated with breast pain and nodularity in women with 'fibrocystic changes' of the breast. When methylxanthine-containing foods and beverages were eliminated from the diet, many women found that the symptomatology resolved. Subsequent studies failed to demon-

strate either of these findings. It is questionable as to whether there is any benefit in requesting that patients eliminate methylxanthines from their diet.

TREATMENT OF MASTALGIA (Figure 3.1)

General

Patients with severe mastalgia should be symptomatic for approximately 6 months prior to considering medical therapy. Patients who are using oral contraceptives or hormone replacement therapy may have resolution of the pain when the hormones are changed or stopped. If the patient wishes to continue using oral contraceptives, she may try a pill with a higher progestogen content. There is no benefit seen with diuretic therapy in the treatment of breast pain, since there is no correlation between total body water and breast pain. Vitamins E, B_1 and B_6 have not been found to be beneficial in the treatment of breast pain. It has been suggested that wearing an exercise sports bra may be helpful in reducing mastalgia. Recent data suggest that dietary modulation and molecular iodine may be useful in the treatment of breast pain. The three most commonly used drug treatments for mastalgia are evening primrose oil, danazol and bromocriptine; these are described in detail later.

Low fat diet

There have been uncontrolled studies which have suggested that a reduction in fat content in the diet resulted in a reduction of cyclical breast pain. Boyd *et al.* conducted a randomized controlled trial to determine whether a reduction in dietary fat along with an increase in complex carbohydrate consumption was associated with a reduction in cyclical breast pain. The study contained 21 patients with severe cyclical mastalgia who had been symptomatic for at least 5 years. Patients were randomized into intervention and control groups. The control group received counseling on the principles of a healthy diet and the intervention group was taught to

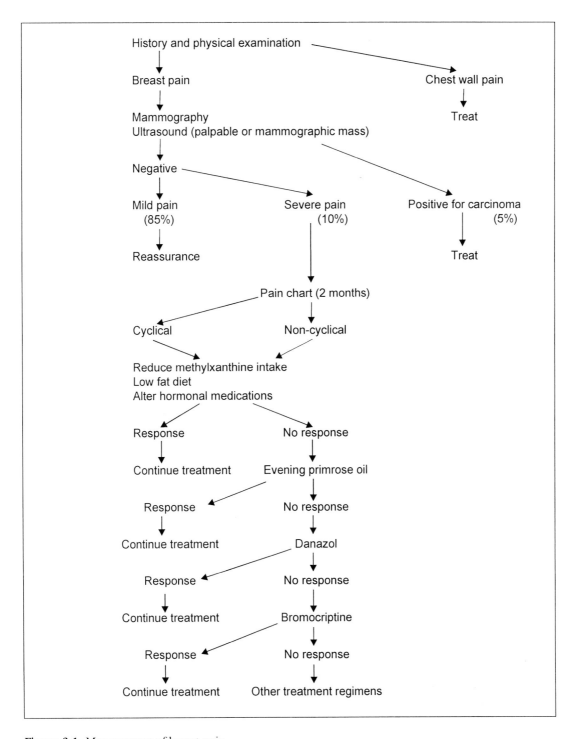

Figure 3.1 Management of breast pain

reduce their fat intake to 15% and increase their carbohydrate intake to 65% of their total caloric intake. Patients were then followed for a total of 6 months. All patients maintained daily records of the breast pain and its association with the menstrual cycle. There was a significant reduction in breast discomfort in the intervention group when compared with patients in the control arm. The authors caution that there is no way to determine whether the improvement in symptoms was due to dietary modulation or placebo effect. They also state that this type of dietary manipulation should be performed under medical supervision, to ensure that the patient does not develop nutritional deficiencies.

Evening primrose oil

Evening primrose oil is a natural product and is a rich source of the essential fatty acid, gamma-linolenic acid. It is a useful alternative when a patient is not interested in using hormonal agents for the treatment of mastalgia. The mechanism of action of evening primrose oil is not understood, but it may act through prostaglandin pathways. Up to 58% of patients with cyclical mastalgia and up to 38% of patients with non-cyclical mastalgia had improvement in their symptoms with evening primrose oil when it was used as the initial treatment. When it was used as second-line treatment, it was successful in 41% of patients with cyclical mastalgia and in 33% of patients with non-cyclical mastalgia. The recommended dosage is 1000 mg three times per day. The onset of improvement is slow and it is recommended that it should be used for 4 months before the treatment is considered a failure. If it is effective in reducing breast pain, evening primrose oil should be continued for a total of 12 months and then stopped. The pain may recur in approximately half of the patients but is usually not severe enough to warrant re-treatment. There are minimal side-effects and the one most commonly reported is abdominal bloating. Only 4% of patients complain of significant adverse effects.

Danazol

Danazol inhibits pituitary gonadotropins and has androgenic, anti-estrogenic and anti-progestogenic activities. There is also a suggestion that there may be a direct effect on breast tissue. When used as the initial treatment, 79% of patients with cyclical breast pain and 40% of patients with non-cyclical mastalgia had improvement in their symptoms. As a second-line treatment, similar percentages of patients responded in each group. Danazol is usually started at a dose of 100 mg twice per day. If a response is observed at 2 months, the dose is reduced to 100 mg per day. If the response is maintained at the lower dose, it is continued for another 2–4 months. The dosage can be further reduced to 100 mg every other day or daily for the last 2 weeks of the menstrual cycle. Treatment is generally discontinued after 6 months. The pain may recur but it is usually not as severe. The major drawback to danazol is the higher rate of side-effects, which include weight gain, menstrual irregularity, headache, nausea and vomiting, acne and abdominal bloating. Thirty per cent of patients complained of significant adverse effects, and in 15% the symptoms were so severe that therapy was discontinued. Due to the higher incidence of side-effects, it is generally recommended that danazol be used as second-line therapy after evening primrose oil has proven to be ineffective.

Bromocriptine

Bromocriptine inhibits the release of prolactin by the pituitary gland and stimulates dopamine receptors in the brain. Prolactin stimulates the glandular tissue of the breast and it is theorized that bromocriptine reduces prolactin production which leads to a reduction in breast pain. When used as the initial treatment, 54% of patients with cyclical breast pain and 33% of patients with non-cyclical mastalgia had improvement in their symptoms. When used as second-line therapy, 46% of patients with cyclical mastalgia and 27% of patients with non-cyclical mastalgia responded. Bromocriptine is started at a dose of 1.25 mg at night. The dose is increased to 2.5 mg twice per day over a 2-week period or longer, depending on adverse effects. The most commonly reported adverse effects are nausea and vomiting, headache and postural hypotension. Constipation, dyspepsia, vasospasm and depression were seen much less frequently. Thirty-five per cent of patients reported significant adverse effects, and in 21% the toxicities were so severe that the treatment was stopped.

Other treatments

Two studies evaluated the effects of aqueous molecular iodine on breast pain in over 1400 women ranging in age from 11 to 87. Patients were treated with molecular iodine with the dosage based upon body weight for a period of 6–9 months. In one study, there were treatment and placebo arms. Response rates varied between 65–72% for those patients treated with iodine and 33% for patients treated with placebo. There was also a second protocol where the molecular iodine was administered either as initial therapy or as the second phase of a cross-over study after receiving a different initial regimen. There were 145 patients in the cross-over study and 74.5% had complete resolution of their breast pain. In the 108 patients treated with molecular iodine alone, 98% of them were without breast pain at the time of study evaluation. Approximately 10% of women experienced toxicity from the treatment which included increased pain (5.7%) and acne (1.1%). There did not appear to be a significant effect on thyroid function, with only 0.4% of patients having thyroid toxicity.

Gestrinone is a synthetic 19-norsteroid which has androgenic, anti-estrogenic and anti-progestagenic properties and has been studied in the treatment of cyclical mastalgia. In a randomized double-blinded study, patients were treated with 2.5 mg gestrinone or placebo twice per week for 3 months. Eighty-nine per cent of the patients in the treatment arm rated the effectiveness as excellent or good compared with only 19% of the patients in the placebo arm. Only 4% of the patients receiving gestrinone reported no improvement in symptoms. Toxicities were reported in 41% of the treatment group and included greasy skin/hair, hirsutism, acne, intermenstrual bleeding, voice change, reduced libido, headache, nausea and reduction in breast size. In patients who wish to avoid pregnancy and are using gestrinone, no other contraceptive is necessary.

Tamoxifen functions as an anti-estrogen within the breast and was studied in a double-blind randomized cross-over trial as a treatment for severe breast pain. Patients with either cyclical or non-cyclical severe mastalgia of 6 months or greater duration were eligible for the study. Patients were randomized to receive either 20 mg of tamoxifen or placebo daily for 3 months, after which those patients who did not respond were then given the alternative treatment. Seventy-one per cent of patients treated with tamoxifen responded favorably, while only 38% responded to placebo. The major toxicities seen with tamoxifen were hot flashes and vaginal discharge. Caution must be used when administering tamoxifen for the treatment of breast pain, since it has been associated with an increased risk for endometrial cancer.

Gonadotropin-releasing hormone analogs, such as goserelin, have been shown to be effective in 81% of patients with severe or refractory cyclical and non-cyclical mastalgia. Widespread use of these agents is hampered by toxicities which include hot flashes, depression, vaginal atrophy, decreased libido and loss of trabecular bone. They are generally used for no longer than 3 months in refractory cases of breast pain.

It has been proposed that breast pain might be associated with an excess of local prostaglandins. Studies have been performed which evaluated the effects of non-steroidal anti-inflammatory agents such as nimesulide. In one report, patients were treated with 100 mg of oral nimesulide twice per day for 15 days, with 70% of the patients having a good to excellent response. The major toxicity was mild gastrointestinal upset and was generally well tolerated.

Surgery is generally not recommended for breast pain, since there is no guarantee for pain relief. Excision of a specific area within the breast where the pain is localized, a trigger spot, will result in a 20% failure rate.

Bibliography

Boyd NF, Shannon P, Kviukov V, *et al.* Effects of a low fat high carbohydrate diet on symptoms of cyclical mastopathy. *Lancet* 1988;2:128–32

Devitt JE. Benign breast disease in the post-menopausal woman. *World J Surg* 1989;13: 731–5

Gateley CA, Maddox PR, Mansel RE, *et al.* Mastalgia refractory to drug treatment. *Br J Surg* 1990;77: 1110–12

Gateley CA, Miers M, Mansel RE, *et al.* Drug treatments for mastalgia: 17 years experience in the Cardiff mastalgia clinic. *J R Soc Med* 1992;85: 12–15

Ghent WR, Eskin BA, Low DA, *et al.* Iodine replacement in fibrocystic disease of the breast. *Can J Surg* 1993;36:453–9

Holland PA, Gateley CA. Drug therapy of mastalgia. What are the options? *Drugs* 1994; 48: 709–16

Maddox PR, Mansel R. Management of breast pain and nodularity. *World J Surg* 1989;13: 699–705

Pain JA, Cahill CJ. Management of cyclical mastalgia. *Br J Clin Pharmacol* 1990; 44: 454–6

Clinical breast evaluation and management of a palpable breast mass

4

L. Jardines

There are several things a woman can do to maintain her breast health, including performing a monthly breast self-examination, clinical breast evaluation and, if age-appropriate, undergoing screening mammography. The clinical breast evaluation includes a detailed history which contains risk factors for breast cancer and a thorough breast examination in the asymptomatic patient. When the woman is presenting with a breast complaint, a detailed history is added to the evaluation. The clinical breast examination is an extremely important part of the physical examination and the primary care physician should have the expertise to feel completely comfortable in performing it. In 1996, the American Cancer Society recommended that women between the ages of 20–40 should have a clinical breast examination every 3 years. For women over the age of 40 years, a clinical breast examination is recommended annually (Table 4.1).

The clinical breast examination should begin with a careful history not only of the presenting problem but also any risk factors for breast cancer which may be relevant to that patient. If she has a complaint, she should be carefully questioned concerning the onset and evolution. Breast cancer can present in a variety of ways and it is extremely important to keep this in mind when taking a history. If a mass has been discovered, it is important to know when it was first discovered and whether it has changed, the size, shape, texture and whether it is mobile or fixed. She should be questioned as to whether she has noted skin changes (edema or retraction). Breast cancer may also present as a change in the nipple and may be manifested by retraction, erosion or discharge. The patient may present with breast pain which is most often of a benign etiology, but in approximately 5% of cases may be the initial presentation of a primary breast malignancy. The patient should be questioned carefully to determine whether the pain is cyclical or non-cyclical, unilateral and focal or bilateral and diffuse. Breast pain associated with an underlying breast cancer is generally localized, non-radiating and is often described as a stabbing pain. In the face of breast pain where the mammogram is normal and there are no physical findings, it is unlikely that there is any serious underlying breast pathology. Occasionally, a patient with breast cancer may present with the complaint of axillary adenopathy. Either axillary pain or upper extremity edema is a particularly ominous presentation of breast cancer.

Table 4.1 American Cancer Society breast screening guidelines

	Age (years)	*Interval*
Breast self-examination	≥20	monthly
Clinical breast examination	20 to 39	every 3 years
	≥40	yearly
Mammography	≥40	yearly

BREAST CANCER RISK FACTORS (Table 4.2)

Gender

Breast cancer is primarily a disease of women; however, it is important to remember that men can also be affected. The ratio of the disease in women versus men is approximately 100:1.

Age

The incidence of breast cancer increases with increasing age and begins to rise at a significant rate at approximately the age of 35 years. Approximately 60% of breast cancer cases are seen in women aged 60 years and older. Breast cancer does occur in young women but is not common. For women who are age 20, the risk of developing breast cancer in the next 10 years is 1 in 2500 whereas for a woman who is 60, the risk is 1 in 29 for the same time period.

Family and medical history

The overall relative risk for breast cancer in women with a positive family history in a first-degree relative is 1.7. It is necessary to determine the number of first- and second-degree family members affected with the disease. In addition, the patient should be questioned concerning the age at which the family member was affected with the disease and whether the disease was unilateral or bilateral. When the first-degree family member has been affected by premenopausal, unilateral breast cancer, the risk is threefold as opposed to bilateral disease where the risk increases to ninefold. When the diagnosis is made in a postmenopausal first-degree family member, the relative risk is increased by 1.5 and when it is bilateral the risk increases fivefold.

If there is a high incidence of premenopausal, bilateral breast cancer in a woman's family she should be questioned also concerning the incidence of ovarian and prostate cancer, since the patient could be at risk for hereditary breast cancer secondary to mutations in either the *BRCA1* or *BRCA2* genes. Families

Table 4.2 Breast cancer risk factors

- Gender
- Age
- Family history
- Previous history of breast cancer
- Age at menarche
- Age at first full-term pregnancy
- Age at menopause
- Pathology from previous breast biopsies
- Alcohol consumption
- History of chest wall irradiation
- ? Exogenous hormone use

with mutations in *BRCA1* have a high incidence of breast, ovarian and prostate cancers while those with altered *BRCA2* have a high incidence of breast cancer and other malignancies. These genes are transmitted in autosomal dominant fashion; therefore, the mutated gene can be inherited through either the maternal or paternal chromosomes and a careful family history is necessary to determine whether the pedigree is consistent with hereditary breast cancer. It was originally reported that women with alterations in *BRCA1* had an 80% chance of developing breast cancer by age 85 and a 60% chance of developing ovarian cancer. However, recent data suggest that the risk for developing breast cancer in the face of a *BRCA1* mutation may not be quite that high and there may be other factors associated with the degree of gene penetrance. Most likely, there are also other genes which are associated with hereditary breast cancer that have not yet been identified.

The majority of authors agree that there is no increased risk for breast cancer when only a second-degree relative, aunt, cousin, or grandmother, has had breast cancer. Most women who develop breast cancer have no family history of the disease. A personal history of breast cancer is also a significant risk for the subsequent development of a second breast cancer and has been estimated to be as high as 1% per year from the time of diagnosis of the initial breast cancer.

The diagnosis of proliferative breast disorders after breast biopsy has also been associated with an increased breast cancer risk and include: hyperplasia, atypical hyperplasia (ductal or lobular) and lobular carcinoma *in situ*. It has been noted that there is only a slightly increased risk (×1.5–2) for developing breast cancer when the diagnosis of either moderate or florid hyperplasia without atypia has been made. There is a moderately increased risk (×4–5) when a diagnosis of atypical hyperplasia has been made. In patients who have a diagnosis of lobular carcinoma *in situ*, there is an ×8–10 elevation in the risk for developing a subsequent invasive breast cancer.

Menstrual and reproductive factors

Early menarche (before age 12) has been associated with a modest risk in breast cancer risk (twofold or less) and the effect decreases with age. Women who undergo menopause before the age of 30 have a two-fold reduction in the breast cancer risk when compared to women who undergo menopause after age 55 years. A first full-term pregnancy before the age of 30 appears to have a protective effect, while a late first full-term pregnancy may be associated with a higher breast cancer risk. There is also a suggestion that lactation provides protection against breast cancer development.

Exogenous hormone use

The data concerning oral contraceptives and hormone replacement therapy (HRT) on breast cancer risk are controversial, and it is unclear whether the prolonged use of oral contraceptives or the use of oral contraceptives before a first full-term pregnancy add to breast cancer risk. A recent study suggested that a woman's risk for breast cancer is slightly increased while she is using oral contraceptives and the risk persists for 10 years after she stops using birth control pills. The authors state that they are unsure whether this small but real increased incidence of breast cancer is related to the oral contraceptives themselves or the breast cancer is being identified earlier, since women using oral contraceptives are followed closely.

Two studies have been published recently which evaluated the effects of HRT on breast cancer risk. In one study, there was a small but statistically significant increase in the incidence of breast cancer, particularly in older women (aged 60–64) who used HRT for longer than 5 years. A second study where women aged 50–64 years were treated with HRT for 8 or more years was associated with an increase in breast cancer risk. Since there are conflicting data concerning breast cancer risk and HRT, patients should be counseled concerning the current state of knowledge in this area. In addition, a detailed risk assessment should be performed concerning their own risk factors for cardiovascular disease and osteoporosis as well as breast, colon and endometrial cancers. By doing so, the patient and her physician will be able to develop an appropriate course of action.

Alcohol use

There appears to be an association between moderate alcohol intake (two drinks/day) and a modest increase in breast cancer risk.

Radiation exposure

An increased rate of breast cancer was noted in survivors of the atomic bomb explosion with a peak latent time of 15–20 years. More recently, patients with Hodgkin's disease treated with mantle irradiation have been noted to have an increased incidence of breast cancer.

PRESENTATION OF BREAST CANCER

With the increasing use of mammography, many breast cancers are detected solely by mammography. When symptoms or signs are present, the most common presenting complaint is a lump within the breast and, depending on the study, this can range from 65 to 76% of cases. Pain is the presenting symptom in approximately 5% of patients, breast enlargement in 1%, skin or nipple retraction in approximately 5%, nipple discharge in about 2%, nipple crusting or erosion in 1%. Approximately 2% of

Table 4.3 Presentation of breast cancer on clinical breast examination

- Breast mass
- Skin/nipple retraction
- Nipple discharge
- Nipple erosion
- Breast pain
- Axillary adenopathy
- Edema of the upper extremity
- Skin edema (peau d'orange)
- Axillary pain

Table 4.4 The seven Ps for clinical breast examination

- Position
- Perimeter
- Palpation
- Pressure
- Pattern of search
- Practice with feedback
- Plan of action

patients with breast cancer will present with axillary adenopathy. In the majority of instances, the tumors are discovered by the patient and this accounts for 70% of all tumors discovered (Table 4.3).

TECHNIQUE OF CLINICAL BREAST EXAMINATION

Clinical breast examination must be performed properly and includes the regional lymph node bearing areas (supraclavicular, infraclavicular, and axillary lymph nodes) and a complete breast examination. The American Cancer Society advocates using the 'seven Ps' in performing the clinical breast examination which include: (1) positions for examination, (2) the perimeter or location of breast tissue, (3) palpation technique with pads of the fingertips, (4) pressure application for breast palpation, (5) pattern of search, (6) practice with feedback from the patient and (7) a plan of action should an abnormality be identified (Table 4.4).

The patient is first observed in a sitting position to observe for asymmetry between the breasts, nipple retraction or skin dimpling (Figure 4.1). The supraclavicular and infraclavicular nodes are examined. To examine each axilla, the patient's arm is supported by the contralateral hand of the examiner to relax the pectoral muscles (Figure 4.2). The ipsilateral hand of the examiner is then used to carefully palpate the axilla. If any nodes are palpated, the size and number should be noted. In addition,

it is important to note whether they are matted or fixed. Next, other maneuvers which can enhance the examiner's ability to detect nipple or skin retraction are asking the patient to press her hands against her hips, lean forward and raise her arms behind and above her head while still in a sitting position (Figures 4.3, 4.4 and 4.5). With the patient sitting in the upright position and her hands behind her head, the upper half of the breast can also be palpated. When she raises her arms above her head, a bimanual examination of the breast can be performed. The patient is then asked to lie in the recumbent position with the head of the examining table elevated at approximately 15 degrees and place the ipsilateral arm above the head (Figure 4.6). A small pillow can be placed behind the shoulder. Patients with extremely large breasts can be asked to rotate their upper body to bring the majority of the breast tissue over the chest wall (Figure 4.7). Breast tissue extends from the clavicle to the sternum to the upper border of the rectus to the latissimus dorsi and this entire area should be examined carefully (Figure 4.8). Breast palpation should be performed using the fingertips, since they are the most sensitive portion of the fingers. During the course of the examination, the amount of pressure applied to each area should be varied, since light pressure will detect lesions close to the surface and deep pressure will detect lesions close to the chest wall. There are many techniques described for performing a breast palpation (Figure 4.9); however, the most important thing is to do the breast examination consistently. If a mass is detected, the size,

Figures 4.1–4.9 are reproduced with permission from: *Clinical Breast Examination: Proficiency Criteria and Guidelines.* **The American Cancer Society, California Division, Breast Health Work Group of the Public Education Committee, February 1988**

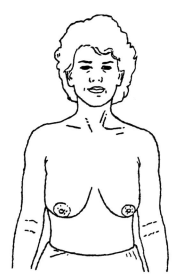

Figure 4.1 The patient should be disrobed from the waist up and the exam should be performed with good lighting

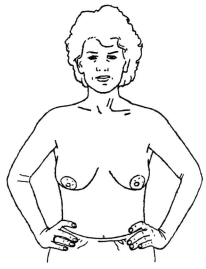

Figure 4.3 The patient should place her hands on her hips and press very hard. The breasts should be inspected for skin or nipple retraction

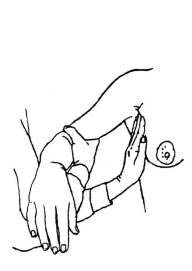

Figure 4.2 Examine the supraclavicular, infra-clavicular and axillary lymph nodes. This demon-strates the proper position to examine the axilla

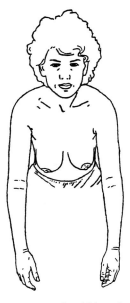

Figure 4.4 The patient should lean forward to look for skin or nipple retraction

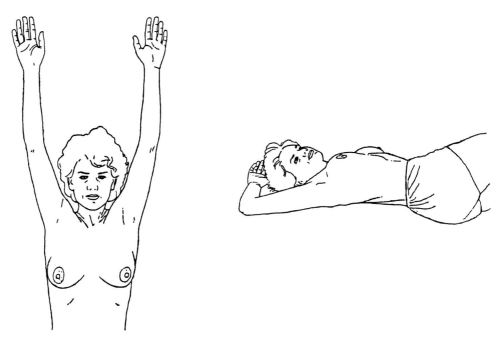

Figure 4.5 The hands should be raised above the head to look for skin or nipple retraction as well as to view the underside of the breast

Figure 4.7 For patients with large breasts, a 45 degree tilt may be an aid in complete breast palpation

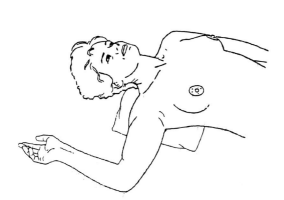

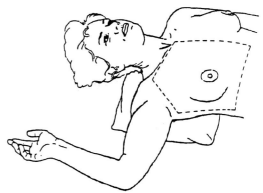

Figure 4.6 The patient should then lie supine. A pillow can be placed behind the ipsilateral shoulder to provide elevation of the chest or the exam table can be raised approximately 15 degrees

Figure 4.8 The perimeter describes the location and extent of breast tissue

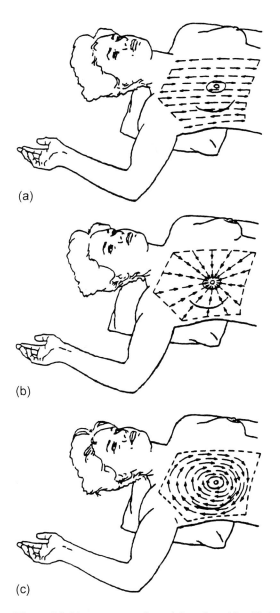

Figure 4.9 Many patterns of search have been identified: (a) the vertical strip; (b) the wedge; (c) the circular pattern

location, consistency and degree of fixation should all be noted. In addition, a plan should be developed to determine the nature of the mass. It is also helpful to reinforce the technique of examination with the patient, so that she may become more comfortable with performing breast self-examination on a monthly basis.

MANAGEMENT OF A PALPABLE BREAST MASS

Most breast masses are due to fibroadenomas, cysts, fibrocystic changes or breast cancer. A fibroadenoma is the most common solid breast mass and is more commonly found in younger women (<25 years of age). Masses secondary to fibrocystic changes are also more common in younger women. Breast cysts become more common in the fourth decade of life and it is impossible to distinguish a benign breast cyst from a solid mass solely on the basis of physical examination. The incidence of breast cancer starts to increase dramatically around the age of 35 years.

It is estimated that there will be approximately 510 new breast cancer cases in women between 20–29 years, 8700 new breast cancer cases in women aged between 30–39 years and 33 400 new breast cancer cases in women between 40–49 years of age over the course of one year, which in 1996, accounts for 0.3%, 4.7% and 18.1%, respectively, of all new breast cancer cases in the United States. The incidence of breast cancer peaks in the 70–79-year-old age group and accounts for 44 700 cases or 24.3% (see Table 4.5). Therefore, the likelihood that a breast mass is secondary to an underlying malignancy increases with age. The possibility that a breast mass in a young woman is secondary to an underlying breast malignancy is small but not zero; therefore, a breast mass in a woman of any age should be evaluated.

The approach to a breast mass varies according to the age of the patient. If a woman of any age has a discrete, dominant breast mass, it requires further evaluation either by ultrasound or aspiration to determine whether it is solid or

Table 4.5 Estimated new breast cancer cases in women by age in 1996

Age	Estimate	Percentage of total
20–29	510	0.3
30–39	8700	4.7
40–49	33 400	18.1
50–59	30 900	16.8
60–69	40 000	21.7
70–79	44 700	24.3
80+	26 000	14.1
Total	184 300	100.0

Table 4.6 Modified triple test

- Clinical breast examination
- Ultrasound directed to palpable mass
- Fine needle aspiration cytology

cystic (fluid-filled). The advantage of ultrasound prior to aspiration is that ultrasound will distinguish a solid from a cystic lesion and then further management can be planned based upon that knowledge (Figure 4.10). It is also possible to differentiate between a benign simple cyst and a complex cyst with ultrasonography. If aspiration is performed and no fluid is obtained, this does not rule out a fluid-filled lesion, since some cysts may have extremely thick walls and may be difficult to aspirate. In addition, if mammography is obtained after aspiration, architectural distortion may be seen on the mammogram secondary to the trauma of the needle, possibly resulting in a false-positive study.

Palpable cystic breast lesions should be aspirated to establish that the cyst is indeed benign and to allow complete evaluation of all the tissue on breast examination. In addition, some breast cysts are extremely painful and aspiration provides symptomatic relief. When intracystic papillary structures are seen on ultrasonography, it may be more prudent to recommend excision of the cyst rather than aspiration due to concern over an intracystic carcinoma. If the fluid obtained from the cyst is bloody or the mass does not resolve completely after aspiration, the patient should undergo mammography and excision of the mass. The bloody fluid can be sent for cytology and if the results are suspicious or conclusive for malignancy, it is then possible to discuss treatment options for breast cancer with the patient. If she is interested in breast conservation, a lumpectomy or partial mastectomy can be performed rather than excisional biopsy as the initial surgical procedure. When the fluid obtained is non-bloody and the mass resolves completely after aspiration, the fluid can be discarded and the patient seen for follow-up, since the incidence of cyst carcinoma is extremely low. If the cyst recurs, the patient should be sent for mammography and a surgical consultation. At this point, it may become necessary to excise a cyst which occurs after repeated aspirations due to concerns of an underlying breast malignancy. Another alternative to excising a recurrent breast cyst is to obtain a pneumocystogram. This is a procedure performed by the radiologist where the cyst is aspirated and air is then injected into the cyst cavity. The patient is then sent for mammography so that the wall of the cyst can be evaluated radiographically. A cyst with irregular walls or intracystic papillary projections should always be removed surgically.

In premenopausal patients where the mass or thickening is questionable, the patient should return to the office for re-examination on days 5–10 of her menstrual cycle. If the mass has resolved, routine screening can then be recommended and if it has not, the patient requires further evaluation. Postmenopausal women with a breast mass or thickening or premenopausal patients with a persistent breast mass require further evaluation.

In young women (<35 years old) with a solid breast mass it is quite reasonable to proceed with a 'modified triple test' which includes breast ultrasound directed towards the palpable abnormality, a clinical breast examination and fine needle aspiration for cytology (Table 4.6). Ultrasonography is recommended as the initial breast imaging modality in this setting since mammography is rarely useful as a screening

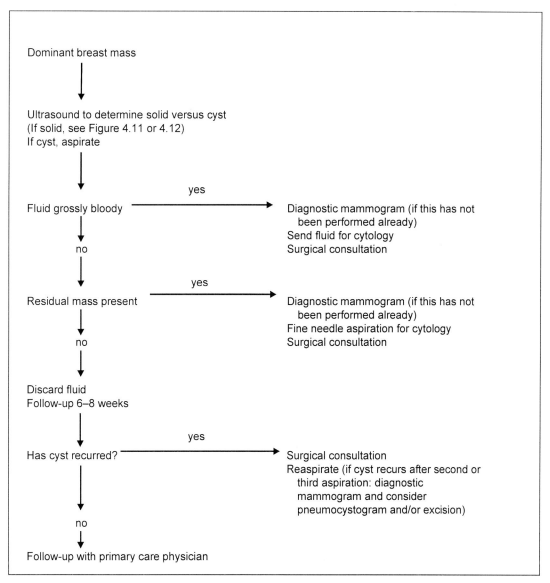

Figure 4.10 Management of a breast cyst

tool in young women. However, it is important to remember that ultrasound should not be used to screen the entire breast but should be directed towards the palpable finding. If any of these tests produces suspicious results, mammography and excision is recommended. Fine needle aspiration cytology is the most sensitive portion of the modified triple test with respect to distinguishing a benign from a malignant process. If all three arms of the modified triple test are consistent with a benign process, follow-up can safely be offered to the patient as an alternative to excision (Figure 4.11).

Some surgeons recommend excision of all solid breast masses, no matter what the etiology and despite the young age of the patient. When making this type of recommendation, it is important to keep in mind that approximately

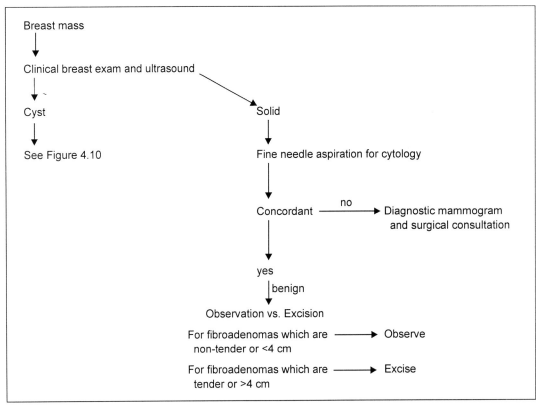

Figure 4.11 Management of a breast mass in women aged <35 years

two-thirds of women who present to specialty breast clinics for evaluation are under 40 years of age. In addition, up to 97% of all breast masses which are excised in young women are benign. Furthermore, approximately 50% of fibroadenomas may decrease in size spontaneously and 16% will remain stable whereas only 32% will increase in size. Therefore, the recommendation of routine excision of all solid breast masses in young women may not be the wisest use of health care resources. For women under the age of 35 where the modified triple test suggests a benign fibroadenoma, the author recommends excision if the mass is large at the time of presentation (>4 cm), it is enlarging, is painful or if the woman requests excision. Breast masses in this age group do require evaluation, however, since there is a small risk of breast cancer in this patient population.

Premenopausal women older than 35 years with a dominant breast mass and post-menopausal women with a persistent solid breast mass or thickening should undergo evaluation, since the incidence of breast cancer begins to rise at the age of 35 and increases steadily through the 70s (Figure 4.12). There have been different methods suggested to approach a solid breast mass in this subset of women. The triple test, which includes mammography, clinical breast examination and fine needle aspiration for cytology has been advocated in evaluating solid breast lesions (Table 4.7). Those who argue for the triple test report that if all three components are concordant there is 100% sensitivity when each element is interpreted as malignant and 100% specificity when each element is interpreted as benign. When there are non-concordant cases,

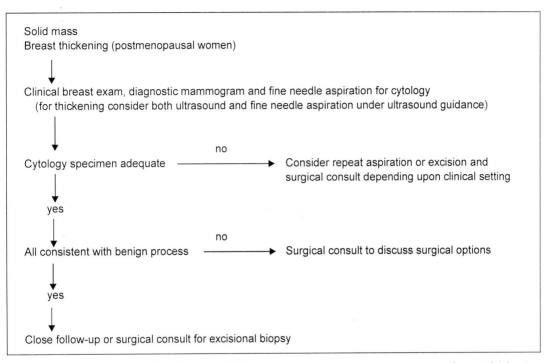

Figure 4.12 Management of a palpable solid breast mass in women aged >35 years or breast thickening in postmenopausal woman

fine needle aspiration cytology is the most predictive element. In a study by Vetto *et al.*, there were no missed cancers and no false-positive malignant diagnoses when the triple test was employed. It is important to keep in mind that there is a learning curve when performing fine needle aspiration for cytology, and a skilled cytopathologist is required to evaluate the test. The advantage to following the guidelines set forth by the triple test is that many breast biopsies for benign disease can be avoided. The disadvantage is that although the incidence of false-negative cytology reports is low in many studies, it is not zero. Therefore, caution must be applied when a decision is made to observe a solid breast mass in an older woman. Others advocate mammography and excision when a

solid breast mass has been identified which will reduce the likelihood of missing a breast cancer to zero. The other alternative is to offer the triple test to the patient and use the results to guide the extent of surgery. In patients where the likelihood of malignancy is low, excisional biopsy of the mass can be recommended. For patients where the likelihood of malignancy is high, treatment options for breast cancer can be discussed and definitive surgical therapy can be undertaken from the outset.

Table 4.7 Triple test

- Clinical breast examination
- Bilateral mammography
- Fine needle aspiration cytology

Bibliography

American Cancer Society. *Breast Cancer Facts and Figures 1996*. American Cancer Society, 1996

American Cancer Society, California Division, Breast Health Work Group of the Public Education Committee. *Clinical Breast Examination. Proficiency Criteria and Guidelines*. California: American Cancer Society, California Division Inc., 1710 Webster Street, Oakland CA 94612, February 1988

Brand IR, Sapherson DA, Brown TS. Breast imaging in women under 35 with symptomatic breast disease. *Br J Radiol* 1993;66:394–7

Colditz GA, Hankinson SE, Hunter DJ, *et al.* The use of estrogens and progestins and the risk of breast cancer in postmenopausal women. *N Engl J Med* 1995;332:1589–93

Ford D, Easton DE, Bishop DT, *et al.* Risk of cancer in *BRCA1* mutation carriers. *Lancet* 1994;343:692–5

Leitch AM, Dodd GD, Constanza M, *et al.* American Cancer Society guidelines for the early detection of breast cancer: update 1997. *CA A Cancer J Clin* 1997;47:150–3

Morrow M. Clinical evaluation. In Harris JR, Lippmann ME, Morrow M, Hellman S, eds. *Diseases of the Breast*. Philadelphia, New York: Lippincott-Raven Publishers. 1995;67–70

Palmer ML, Tsangaris TN. Breast biopsy in women 30 years old or less. *Am J Surg* 1993;165:708–12

Rosen PP. Proliferative breast 'disease'. An unresolved diagnostic dilemma. *Cancer* 1993;71:3798–807

Stanford JL, Weiss NS, Voigt LF, *et al.* Combined estrogen and progestin hormone replacement therapy in relation to risk of breast cancer in middle-age women. *J Am Med Assoc* 1995;274:137–42

Struewing JP, Hartage P, Wacholder S, *et al.* The risk of cancer associated with specific mutations of *BRCA1* and *BRCA2* in Ashkenazi Jews. *N Engl J Med* 1997;336:1401–8

Vetto J, Pommier R, Schmidt WA, *et al.* Use of the 'triple test' for palpable breast lesions yields high diagnostic accuracy and cost savings. *Am J Surg* 1995;169:519–22

Vetto JT, Pommier RF, Schmidt WA, *et al.* Diagnosis of palpable breast lesions in younger women by the modified triple test is accurate and cost-effective. *Arch Surg* 1996;131:967–74

Diagnostic imaging of the breast   5

B. Cavanaugh and S.O. Asbell

IMAGING EVALUATION OF THE BREAST

In the last three decades, the field of breast imaging has undergone tremendous growth, with advances and refinement of techniques in mammography, and with the introduction and continued refinement of additional modalities such as ultrasound and magnetic resonance imaging (MRI). Clinical trials have demonstrated the efficacy of screening mammography for early detection of breast cancer, with resultant increased survival and decreased mortality. Ultrasound and MRI have an established role in breast evaluation, and the role of MRI is expanding with current research. As technology advances, increased help from computers – digital mammography and computer-assisted diagnosis – will become available.

As more women obtain screening mammograms, the primary care physician must be able to explain to his/her patients the meaning of the mammography reports. Women want to understand them and need them interpreted. Any reason for the recommendation of additional imaging or need for biopsy must be explained. Even when the radiologist has reviewed the results with the patient, the patient's anxiety may inhibit her from a full discussion of her concerns. In the environment of the trusted primary care physician's office, the patient frequently asks questions and expresses concerns. This chapter will contain sufficient data about breast imaging to assist the primary care physician.

MAMMOGRAPHY

Mammography was first used about 85 years ago, and its usefulness as a screening tool for the early detection of breast cancer was first investigated in the 1950s. In the past, mammography was performed on standard X-ray units, using conventional film. There was appropriate concern over the radiation dose to the breast with this technique. Thus, specialized film-screen cassettes and dedicated X-ray units were developed. This allowed much greater accuracy at a much lower radiation dose to the patient. This, in addition to the early diagnosis of cancers in the screening trials and high degree of successful treatment, led to the acceptance of widespread screening mammography.

Data on the radiosensitivity of breast tissue has been obtained from atomic bomb survivors and from women who had radiation treatments for Hodgkin's disease and those exposed to fluoroscopy for postpartum mastitis. The radioresistance of mature breast tissue, as well as the very low radiation dose of today's mammogram, makes screening mammography (that is, performed on women aged 40 years and over) a low radiation exposure risk. This is further supported by the decreased breast cancer mortality of women who obtain screening mammograms as compared to those who do not.

Terminology in mammography reports can be confusing and frustrating for the clinician faced with a questioning, anxious patient. The American College of Radiology is attempting to standardize terminology in mammography reports, to improve clarity of communication of information to referring physicians as well as to lay the groundwork for a national database for mammography and breast cancer monitoring. This also has a potential application for future computer-assisted diagnosis. A Breast Imaging Reporting and Data System (BI-RADS) with standardized lexicon has been developed.

Technique and instrumentation

Modern, dedicated mammography units differ from conventional X-ray units. The X-ray tubes, screen-film combinations, and positioning techniques are designed to produce high contrast, high resolution images that maximize tissue resolution while minimizing radiation dose to the patient. A mammogram is obtained by compressing the breast between a compression paddle and a tray which holds an X-ray cassette and grid. X-rays pass through the breast, exposing the film in the cassette. Two standard views are obtained: mediolateral oblique and craniocaudad. The resultant film displays densities of differing opacities that correspond to the different types of tissue in the breast: fat density (fat), water density (fibrous and glandular tissue), and calcium. Additional images may be obtained: spot compression views, which compress a smaller area of tissue for better separation of overlying structures; magnification views, which are spot compression views with radiographic magnification, providing better separation and better detail; or views with slightly different positioning such as lateral or rolled craniocaudad views, to better define or to identify the location of an area of interest.

Many women become concerned when additional images are requested. A mammogram is a two-dimensional representation of a three-dimensional structure and artifacts can occur. Most additional imaging is performed to spread out the three-dimensional structures of the breast so that overlapping tissues neither simulate a mass nor hide one.

Screening mammography

As a screening tool for asymptomatic women, properly performed mammography can detect 85–95% of cancers that are not yet palpable. Early detection of breast cancer through screening mammography has been demonstrated to decrease mortality in women aged 50–69 years. There is preliminary evidence that screening will also decrease mortality in women aged 40–49 years. There are few data on screening women older than 70 years; small non-palpable cancers are certainly detected in this age group, but studies to evaluate the effect of screening on breast cancer mortality are not available for women over 70 years.

The American College of Radiology and the American Cancer Society recommend that women begin to obtain screening mammograms at age 40. Recently, the National Cancer Advisory Board has recommended that the National Cancer Institute advise women between 40 and 49 years to have screening mammograms every 1–2 years if they are at average risk for breast cancer. Women who are at higher than average risk should seek medical advice about beginning mammography before age 40 and about the screening frequency while in their 40s. Proper technique and interpretive expertise are critically important in mammography, as will be discussed below.

Screening for breast cancer is unlike other diagnostic studies in that the 'patient' is completely asymptomatic. It involves healthy women and has a low yield of abnormal studies, about five non-palpable invasive cancers found per 1000 women. Techniques in screening mammography must maximize the early detection of cancer with minimal morbidity to women. Scrupulous attention must be made to the quality and maintenance of the mammographic equipment that is used; meticulous positioning technique; optimization of film-screen combinations and specialized developing conditions; attention to the conditions under which the mammograms are viewed and interpreted; appropriate training of the interpreters; and careful auditing of outcomes of a screening practice: all of these parameters have been analyzed, with resulting quality assurance guidelines made widely available. In the United States, adherence to screening guidelines is mandated by law with the implementation of the Mammography Quality Standards Act.

The positive predictive value of mammographic findings is approximately 20–40%, i.e. only two to four of ten suspicious breasts on mammogram will be malignant on either percutaneous or excisional biopsy. A screening practice with an older population, all with prior studies available for comparison, will yield a higher positive predictive value of an abnormal mammogram than a practice with a younger population.

The radiographic appearance of normal breast tissue is extremely variable (Figure 5.1). Mammograms can be nearly completely fatty (a radiolucent background against which abnormal tissue is well seen) or completely radiodense (a background against which abnormal tissue can be obscured) or any combination in between. Normal tissues that may overlie one another when the breast is compressed may produce pseudomasses on the resultant mammogram, or normal tissue may partially or completely obscure a true mass. Specialized images are used for better definition of areas of concern.

On a mammogram, the typical suspicious mass is denser than surrounding tissues, has irregular or spiculated margins, and can be seen on two orthogonal views of the breast (Figure 5.2). The typical benign mass is less dense than surrounding tissues, and has well-circumscribed margins with a round or oval shape (Figure 5.3). Many masses fall somewhere between these two appearances and comprise the large category of 'indeterminate' masses (Figure 5.4). These are of concern because a malignancy can have a subtle mammographic appearance that can be similar to a benign mass. Additional imaging helps to define the degree of suspicion to determine the need for percutaneous or excisional biopsy.

Mammography can visualize tiny calcifications. Benign breast calcifications are common in skin, fibroadenomas, arterial walls, or due to fat necrosis, or micro- or macrocysts (so-called milk of calcium). These often have appearances that are typical for their type and do not present a diagnostic problem. Benign calcification cannot always be distinguished from calcifications within malignant tissue based on their mammographic appearance alone. The detection and analysis of calcifications requires meticulous mammographic technique, and magnification views are needed to characterize accurately the morphology, number, and distribution of the calcifications.

Invasive malignancies frequently contain visible calcifications; of intraductal malignancies, about 75% have calcification as the sole radiographic finding (Figure 5.5). In general, linear or branching calcifications strongly correlate with malignancy, while rounded calcifications of uniform size and density correlate with benign tissue. However, there is considerable overlap in the appearance of benign and malignant calcifications.

Diagnostic mammography

A diagnostic mammogram, in contrast to a screening mammogram, is performed on a symptomatic woman. While mammography is an excellent screening tool, a normal mammogram cannot *exclude* the presence of malignancy. The ultimate assessment of the symptomatic woman rests on the findings at physical examination, with correlation of imaging findings as deemed clinically appropriate.

For a woman over the age of 25–30 years who presents with worrisome changes in the breast, mammography is the primary imaging modality. Clinical findings can include: a palpable mass, thickening, or other area of palpable concern; a suspicious nipple discharge; or suspicious skin changes such as dimpling (including new nipple inversion). The mammogram assesses the radiographic characteristics of the area of concern; a palpable abnormality may be

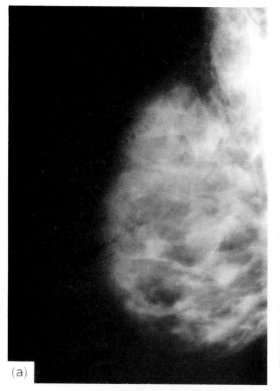

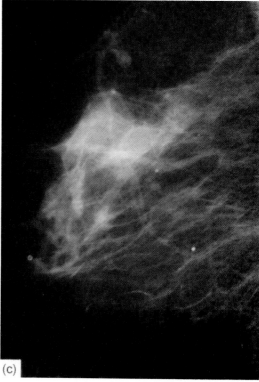

Figure 5.1 Variation in radiographic appearance of normal breast tissue: (a) radiographically dense; (b) fatty (with some typically benign calcifications); (c) scattered fibroglandular opacities

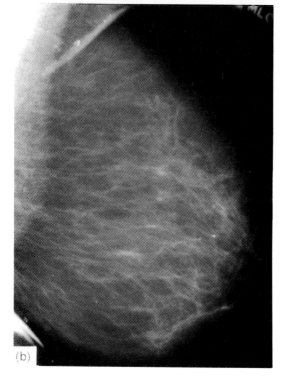

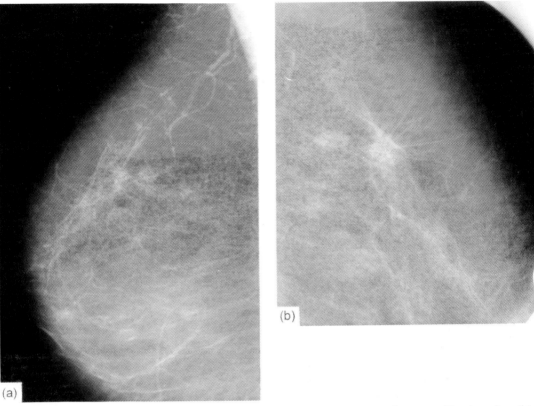

Figure 5.2 Left mediolateral oblique (MLO) view (a) and MLO compression magnification view (b) demonstrating a small spiculated mass in the upper breast: infiltrating ductal carcinoma. The circumscribed oval mass adjacent to this appears benign and was a fibroadenoma

marked with a radio-opaque marker such as a BB so that a close correlation can be made. Ultrasound is often useful for further evaluation, particularly to confirm that a benign appearing mass represents a cyst or sonographically benign solid mass. The mammogram also screens the clinically normal breast tissue for evidence of non-palpable abnormalities that may indicate the presence of multifocal or multicentric disease, or that may be unrelated to the original complaint. While an abnormal mammogram can corroborate clinical findings, a normal mammogram cannot exclude the diagnosis of breast cancer; the ultimate management of palpable abnormalities must be based on the clinical impression.

A woman under 25 years of age presenting with a mass with clinically benign features on palpation can be evaluated first with ultrasound to characterize the mass as cystic or solid. Mammography is usually not indicated in this age group. Even though the radiation dose of mammography is extremely low, there is a theoretical risk to the relatively radiosensitive breast tissue of young women. In addition, the likelihood of detecting breast cancer at this age is extremely low. Thus the risk–benefit ratio does not favor mammography in women under the age of 25 years. In fact, an imaging study may not be necessary; if the patient does not want a palpable mass to remain in her breast, the ultrasonic demonstration of a simple cyst or typically benign solid mass will not obviate an excisional biopsy. These women can proceed directly to a breast surgeon, either for clinically guided aspiration or for excision.

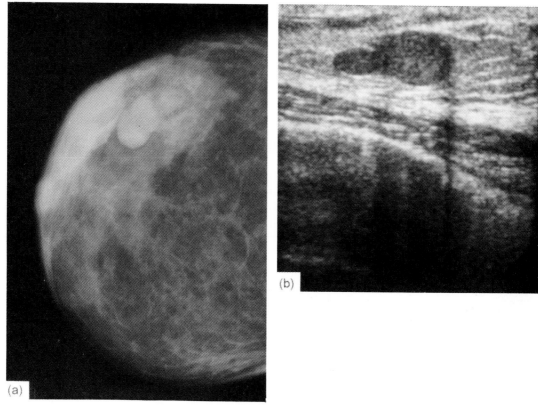

Figure 5.3 Fibroadenoma: right craniocaudal (CC) view (a) demonstrating a primarily circumscribed lobulated mass, with circumscribed margins confirmed on compression magnification views (not shown). Ultrasound of this mass (b) demonstrates benign features: ellipsoid macrolobulated shape, circumscribed margins, uniformly hypoechoic

Mammographic evaluation of the woman with breast cancer

Mammography is useful in the preoperative evaluation of women with known breast cancer who are considering breast conserving surgery. It evaluates for mammographic signs of extent of tumor that may not be appreciated at physical exam. Mammography can also screen the remaining breast tissue in order to detect non-palpable multifocal, multicentric or contralateral disease. These findings are used to evaluate women who are candidates for breast conserving treatment.

Following breast conserving treatment, mammography is valuable for the early detection of recurrence. For women treated with mastectomy, imaging of the mastectomy site or the reconstructed breast has not usually been helpful. Occasionally, nodules develop in a TRAM (transposition of the rectus abdominis muscle) reconstruction due to fat necrosis, and a mammogram can confirm the typical appearance of fat necrosis.

Digital mammography and computer-assisted diagnosis

The term digital mammography includes both the primary acquisition of mammographic images with digital detectors rather than with film-screen cassettes, and the secondary digitization of film-screen mammographic images.

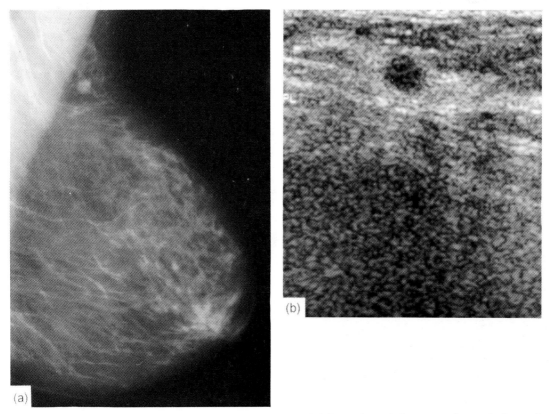

Figure 5.4 Infiltrating ductal carcinoma: left mediolateral oblique view (a) demonstrating an indeterminate mass in upper breast; compression magnification views (not shown) demonstrated indistinct margins. Ultrasound (b) demonstrates a hypoechoic mass with indistinct margins, a suspicious appearance

For both, the goal is computerization of the mammographic image. In conventional film-screen mammography, a film/intensifying screen combination is exposed to an X-ray beam that is directed through the breast; the film-screen image can be digitized and the information stored in a computer. A direct digital mammogram is acquired when the X-ray beam 'exposes' a digital receptor rather than the photographic emulsion on X-ray film.

Digital mammography has several advantages over film-screen mammography. Digital images can be stored compactly and are not subject to degradation from imperfect storage conditions or over time, as is film. Viewing conditions can be controlled more precisely on a computer monitor as compared with a view box, and images can be manipulated to optimize contrast and grayscale. Different types of computer assisted diagnosis are being investigated. The combined effort of a radiologist and computer analysis of digital images has been demonstrated to increase the positive predictive value of positive findings and has potential for decreasing unnecessary biopsies from false-positive mammograms. A digitized image can also be transmitted to another computer, allowing for the possibility of teleradiology, which has important implications for the widespread availability of expert breast imaging.

ULTRASOUND

High resolution real-time ultrasound equipment has not yet been shown to be useful in screening for breast cancer, but it is very useful

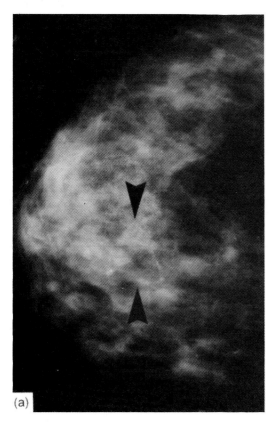

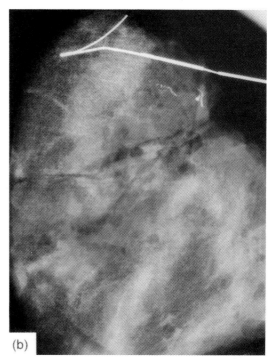

Figure 5.5 Ductal carcinoma *in situ*: right craniocaudal view (a) demonstrating a suspicious cluster of calcifications in the medial breast (arrow); some benign calcifications are scattered in the subareolar and outer breast. Specimen radiograph (b) more clearly shows their pleomorphic and linear morphology

for diagnostic imaging of the breast. In women under 25 years of age who have a palpable mass with clinically benign features and who require an imaging study, this is the study of choice. It is also indicated for the further evaluation of some mammographic findings and often as additional evaluation of a palpable mass in women over 25–30 years. It may be used to evaluate the integrity of breast implants, although it is not as accurate as MRI.

Using strict imaging criteria, ultrasound can clearly distinguish simple cysts from other masses (Figure 5.6). A simple cyst requires no further management unless it is symptomatic. A mass with internal echoes or thick walls or lacking posterior acoustic enhancement may be a benign complex cyst or a solid mass. If the mass is not palpable, such a distinction can be made

by aspirating it with a small gauge needle (from 18 to 25 gauge depending on the cyst) using real-time sonographic guidance.

Ultrasound can assist in the evaluation of solid masses, demonstrating either typically benign features or suspicious features (Figure 5.4). It can also be helpful when assessing other mammographic abnormalities such as areas of asymmetry or questionable findings that are abnormal on one view only. A negative ultrasound does not exclude the presence of malignancy; malignant masses can be isoechoic with adjacent normal tissue, thus becoming invisible to the ultrasound transducer, and intraductal malignancies are often manifest solely by sonographically invisible calcifications.

Color Doppler ultrasound has been investigated for the additional characterization of solid masses. Since malignancy is accompanied by neovascularization, analysis of vascular characteristics can theoretically distinguish benign from malignant masses. However, many cancers are relatively avascular, and many benign masses are hypervascular. Thus, if mammographic findings are indeterminate, a benign Doppler flow analysis is not sufficient to deter biopsy. Therefore the clinical utility of color Doppler analysis has not yet been established.

MAGNETIC RESONANCE IMAGING (MRI)

MRI of the breast has an established role in the evaluation of the integrity of breast implants as well as potential roles in the diagnostic evaluation of the breast. This study is performed with a dedicated breast surface coil: the patient lies prone with her breast suspended in the coil, with some coils using gentle compression. Depending on the indication for the study, intravenous contrast may or may not be used, and pulse sequences are chosen according to the tissue characteristics that the radiologist wishes to examine.

MRI of the breast is the study of choice for the evaluation of breast implants. It allows imaging of the entire implant, unlike mammography and ultrasound which image only the anterior walls of the implants. The integrity of the implant shell is evaluated, and extravasated silicone can be identified.

The role of MRI in the diagnosis and preoperative evaluation of breast cancer is being actively studied. Malignancies consistently enhance following administration of intravenous paramagnetic contrast agents, but some benign tissue enhances as well. The pulse sequences that optimally distinguish benign and malignant tissue have not yet been determined, and different institutions are using different sequences. Studies that attempt to evaluate indeterminate mammography findings, to distinguish benign from malignant tissue in an attempt to decrease the incidence of biopsies, have demonstrated high sensitivity for malignancy but often with low specificity.

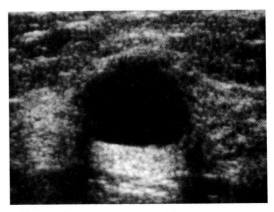

Figure 5.6 Ultrasound appearance of a simple cyst

MRI may have a role in the staging of breast cancer. In women with known breast cancer, it has been able to detect mammographically and clinically occult multifocal and multicentric disease in women thought to be candidates for breast conserving therapy. The usefulness of this information, which potentially influences the choice of breast conserving therapy versus mastectomy, remains to be established. We already know that, for women who are mammographically or clinically lumpectomy candidates (presumably many of whom would have been multicentric on MRI, had it been available), survival is equivalent for women who have mastectomies and women who have breast conserving therapy. It is possible that MRI will identify a subgroup of women who are at high risk for recurrence, thus not so much altering survival but sparing them a second surgery when their cancer recurs.

Eventually, MRI may have a role for breasts that are difficult to evaluate mammographically, either due to radiographically dense tissue or due to the presence of radio-opaque implants, which even with optimal mammographic positioning will inevitably obscure some breast tissue. As the image characteristics that distinguish benign and malignant tissue become more clearly understood, and as the pulse sequences that best display them become optimized, MRI will probably have an invaluable role in breast imaging. At this time, evaluation of implant integrity is the only clinically established role for MRI.

GALACTOGRAPHY

Galactography, the injection of radio-opaque contrast into the mammary ducts, assists in evaluating a source of abnormal discharge. The duct producing the discharge is identified and cannulated with a very thin (27 gauge) needle or cannula. Following the injection of water-soluble contrast into the duct to the point at which the patient senses fullness (usually 0.5–1.0 ml), mammograms using gentle compression are taken. The caliber and contour of the ducts are evaluated and abnormal filling defects identified.

Bibliography

de Lafontan B, Daures JP, Salicru B, *et al.* Isolated clusters of microcalcifications: diagnostic value of mammography – series of 400 cases with surgical verification. *Radiology* 1994;190:479–83

Farria DM, Bassett LW, Kimme-Smith C, *et al.* Mammography quality assurance from A to Z. *Radiographics* 1994;14:371–85

Feig SA, Yaffe MJ. Digital mammography, computer-aided diagnosis, and telemammography. *Radiol Clin N Am* 1995;33:1205–29

Harms SE, Flamig DP, Evans WP, *et al.* MR imaging of the breast: current status and future direction. *Am J Roentgenol* 1994;163:1039–47

Jackson VP. The current role of ultrasonography in breast imaging. *Radiol Clin N Am* 1995;33:1161–70

Mendelsohn EB. Evaluation of the post operative breast. *Radiol Clin N Am* 1992;30:107–38

Sickles EA. Mammographic features of 3000 consecutive breast cancers. *Am J Roentgenol* 1986;146: 661–3

Sickles EA. Periodic follow-up of probably benign lesions: results in 3,184 consecutive cases. *Radiology* 1991;179:463–8

Sickles EA, Ominisky SH, Sollitto RA, *et al.* Medical audit of a rapid throughput mammography screening practice: methodology and results of 27,114 examinations. *Radiology* 1990;175:323–7

Tabar L, Fagerberg G, Duffy SW, *et al.* Update of the Swedish two-county program of mammographic screening for breast cancer. *Radiol Clin North Am* 1992;30:187–210

Interventional breast procedures 6

D.S. Copit and S.O. Asbell

INTRODUCTION

Mammography has always differed from other divisions of diagnostic radiology because it is one of the few fields of radiology where patients return year after year for a study, providing an opportunity for the patient and the mammographer to get to know each other. For some patients, mammographers perform yearly physical breast examinations along with mammographic interpretations, becoming someone whom the patient thinks of as 'her doctor.'

In the USA, the role of the mammographer is evolving with increasing need for direct contact with the patient. Breast imaging includes not only four-view mammograms, but also diagnostic breast evaluation using additional mammographic views such as spot compression and magnification views, breast ultrasound, and sometimes, magnetic resonance imaging. More recently, the breast imager has become involved with other diagnostic breast procedures such as cyst aspiration, fine needle aspiration biopsy (FNAB), and core needle biopsy (CNB) using both sonographic and stereotactic guidance. With the addition of these procedures, the radiologist has also had to accept the added responsibility for patient care and management.

There are three major reasons for the utilization of image-directed core needle biopsy. One is to relieve the anxiety often associated with the delay in scheduling a surgical biopsy in the operating room when an abnormality has been found on mammography. Using this procedure in the X-ray suite may thus provide a concerned patient with a diagnosis, usually within 24 h. Cost containment is a crucial issue. With the cost of the operating room avoided, image-directed core needle biopsies can be more cost-effective. Finally, by eliminating surgical biopsies, scar formation and mammographic pseudolesions which may cause dilemmas with future mammographic interpretation can be avoided.

HISTORY AND DEVELOPMENT OF BREAST PROCEDURES

For suspected tumors found only on X-ray, percutaneous procedures including biopsy and aspiration may be performed by the radiologist. By 1989, image-directed percutaneous breast procedures for mainly impalpable lesions began to be performed and reported by radiologists. These earliest reports used fine needle aspiration biopsy with good results. As of 1990, Parker and colleagues introduced the large core needle biopsy with a 14 gauge needle used under stereotactic guidance. This led to improved accuracy. Ultrasound guidance is now also used with similar accuracy.

TECHNICAL ASPECTS OF CORE NEEDLE BIOPSY

The basic procedure of core needle biopsy is the same whether sonographic or stereotactic guidance is used. The differences between the methods has to do with patient positioning, length of the procedure, and the use of ionizing radiation (stereotactic) or sound waves (ultrasound). Local anesthesia and sterile technique are employed. At least five cores of tissue are obtained; more tissue may be necessary if calcifications are present. With stereotactic guidance, the patient is frequently biopsied in the prone position with the physician and assistant working beneath the patient.

If sonographic guidance is used, the woman lies on her back and her breast is not compressed. The radiologist watches the needle on the screen throughout the procedure. This real-time imaging provides immediate and direct feedback regarding the movement of the needle and its relationship to the lesion as well as to the rest of the breast tissue and chest wall. Because the breast is not in compression and the woman's head is not turned to one side, sonographic guidance is tolerated somewhat better than a stereotactically guided biopsy.

INDICATIONS FOR CORE NEEDLE BIOPSY

Mammographers attempt to place radiographic abnormalities into categories which provide guidance as to the appropriate time interval for a follow-up study or the need for histologic evaluation. For example, lesions which are considered probably benign, such as well-circumscribed masses, clusters of round or oval microcalcifications, and asymmetric fibroglandular densities, can be followed with periodic 6-month follow-up studies until a 2- to 3-year stability is achieved. These lesions do not need to be biopsied unless they change on a subsequent study or if the patient anxiety level is such that she cannot tolerate the follow-up studies. Lesions which are categorized as highly suspicious for malignancy require surgical opinion.

There is a large group of mammographic abnormalities which are considered 'indeterminate' and for which a biopsy should be considered. These lesions fall somewhere between the 'probably benign' and 'highly suspicious' abnormalities and often encompass a diverse group of abnormalities, including partially well circumscribed masses, masses with microlobulated borders, and many different clusters of microcalcifications. While the majority of these lesions are not cancer, there is usually sufficient question to seek a specific diagnosis. These lesions are well suited for a stereotactic or sonographic core needle biopsy.

Many radiologists will not biopsy palpable lesions, as they are usually handled by a breast surgeon; however, this agreement varies from institution to institution. Some surgeons who do not normally refer palpable lesions for imaging-directed biopsy may do so depending on their own time constraints and patient anxiety, as imaging-directed biopsy does not require operating room time and personnel. In fact, one of the major advantages of an imaging-directed biopsy is the ability to perform the biopsy at a moment's notice while ensuring accuracy because of the X-ray guidance provided by direct visualization of the needle path through the lesion.

COMPLICATIONS AND CONTRAINDICATIONS

Complications of core needle biopsy are the formation of a hematoma and infection. Most women experience some degree of bruising following the biopsy, but this can be prevented or limited by the use of firm compression after each sample of tissue is removed from the breast and the use of ice following the procedure. Patients using aspirin or anticoagulants can have biopsies, but it is preferable to adjust these medications to the lowest acceptable dosage to reduce the risk of hematoma formation. In Parker's large multi-center study, only six complications (three infections and three hematomas) were reported. Risk of seeding the tumor tract is low. One case after a core needle biopsy was reported.

FUTURE DIRECTIONS FOR IMAGE-DIRECTED CORE BIOPSY

Increasing numbers of patients should undergo core biopsy of the breast in the future as referring physicians and radiologists become more comfortable with this procedure as an alternative to surgical biopsy. Recent studies have shown, as would be expected, an increase in accuracy of image-directed core biopsy with an increase in experience of the radiologist performing the biopsy. Diagnostic radiologists must be aware of the risk implications if the procedure is not performed properly or lesions are missed.

CYST ASPIRATION

Cyst aspiration under sonographic guidance is a quick, painless procedure when performed with experienced hands. There are three main indications for cyst aspiration: (1) if a patient continues to be concerned about the mass in her breast even when she is reassured that it is a cyst by sonography and definitely benign or because she is concerned because it is causing her tenderness; (2) if the cyst does not fulfill strict criteria for a cyst by sonography, and (3) in order to prove that the mammographic and sonographic abnormality are one and the same. Strict criteria are available for defining a cyst sonographically and for explaining to the patient that most cysts are benign. Cysts such as those with thick walls or poor internal echoes do not fulfill the criteria and require needle aspiration to prove that they are indeed cysts. Some patients are not comfortable knowing that they have a mass in their breast and request aspiration for psychological reasons.

Cyst aspiration is usually performed under local anesthesia with a small gauge needle (from 18 to 25 gauge depending on the cyst) using real-time sonographic guidance.

Bibliography

Crylak D. Induced costs of low-cost screening mammography. *Radiology* 1988;168:661–3

Dowlatsahi K, Gent HJ, Schmidt R, *et al.* Nonpalpable breast tumors: diagnosis with stereotaxic localization and fine needle aspiration. *Radiology* 1989; 170:427–33

Doyle A, Murray K, Nelson E, *et al.* Selective use of image-guided large-core needle biopsy of the breast: accuracy and cost-effectiveness. *Am J Roentgenol* 1995;165:281–4

Evans WP, Cade SH. Needle localization and fine needle aspiration biopsy of nonpalpable breast lesions with use of standard and stereotactic equipment. *Radiology* 1989;173:53–6

Harter LP, Curtis JS, Pronto G, *et al.* Malignant seeding of the needle track during stereotaxic core needle breast biopsy. *Radiology* 1992;185:713–14

Parker SH, Burbank F, Jackman RJ, *et al.* Percutaneous large core breast biopsy: a multi-institutional study. *Radiology* 1991;179:463–8

Parker SH, Jobe WE, Dennis MA, *et al.* US-guided automated large-core breast biopsy. *Radiology* 1993; 187:507–11

Parker SH, Lovin JB, Jobe WE, *et al.* Nonpalpable breast lesions: stereotactic automated large-core biopsies. *Radiology* 1991;180:403–7

Parker SH, Lovin JB, Jobe WE, *et al.* Stereotactic breast biopsy with a biopsy gun. *Radiology* 1990;176: 741

Sickles EA. Periodic follow-up of probably benign mammographic lesions: results of 3184 consecutive cases. *Radiology* 1991;179:463–8

Nipple discharge

7

L. Jardines

INTRODUCTION

Nipple discharge is a common presenting breast complaint in the primary care setting and can be a significant cause of concern for both the patient and the physician providing his or her care. When breast massage or stimulation is performed, approximately 19% of women will produce nipple secretions. Spontaneous nipple discharge, which is less common, is the primary complaint in 3–8% of women who undergo breast surgery. Approximately 10–13% of women and 20% of men who undergo surgery for nipple discharge will have carcinoma as the cause of the nipple discharge.

Nipple discharge is more common in younger women; however, the likelihood that a pathologic nipple discharge will be associated with an underlying carcinoma increases with the age of the patient. Approximately one-third of women older than 60 years of age with spontaneous nipple discharge were diagnosed with breast cancer, while only 7% of women younger than 60 years had a malignancy. The mean age of women with breast carcinoma presenting as nipple discharge was 56 years, with a range of 30–78 years. Bloody nipple discharge without an associated breast mass during pregnancy has been reported and can be managed conservatively.

TYPES OF NIPPLE DISCHARGE

There are three categories of nipple discharge: (1) galactorrhea, (2) physiologic and (3) pathologic.

Galactorrhea is bilateral, milky, involves multiple ducts and is not associated with pregnancy or lactation. It may occur in young girls as they enter puberty and may last for several months to a year without any underlying pathology. Galactorrhea may also be idiopathic or secondary to certain medications, chest wall trauma or endocrine abnormalities. The three most common causes of galactorrhea in women are idiopathic with normal menses, pituitary tumors and idiopathic associated with amenorrhea, in that order. Numerous medications and drugs have been associated with galactorrhea and include oral contraceptives, tricyclic antidepressants, cannabis, antihypertensives and phenothiazines (Table 7.1). Several endocrine disorders including most frequently pituitary adenomas and to a lesser degree thyroid dysfunction may also be associated with galactorrhea.

Physiologic nipple discharge is not spontaneous and may be caused by breast or nipple manipulation when checking for nipple discharge, by exogenous estrogen or by sexual stimulation. It is generally bilateral, serous and arises from multiple ducts. Funderburk and Syphax suggest that when non-spontaneous discharge is serous or bloody and not associated with a mass, a galactogram may be helpful. If the galactogram is negative and nipple cytology is negative, the patient should be re-examined in

Table 7.1 Medications associated with galactorrhea

- Oral contraceptives
- Phenothiazines
- Benzodiazepines
- Isoniazid
- Reserpine

Table 7.2   Pathologic nipple discharge

- Spontaneous
- Unilateral
- Single duct
- Intermittent
- Persistent

Table 7.3   Etiology of pathologic nipple discharge

- Papilloma
- Duct ectasia
- Fibrocystic disease
- Carcinoma
- Other

approximately 3–6 months. If the repeat clinical evaluation is negative, no treatment is offered and the patient should be followed unless the discharge becomes spontaneous.

Pathologic nipple discharge is generally unilateral, localized to a single duct, spontaneous, intermittent and persistent (Table 7.2). The character of the fluid varies and may be bloody, serosanguinous, watery, cloudy, serous or green–gray. No matter what the character of the discharge is from the nipple, the underlying cause is generally benign. The etiologies of pathologic nipple discharge in order of decreasing frequency are an intraductal papilloma and/or papillomatosis (44%), mammary duct ectasia (23%), fibrocystic disease (16%) and carcinoma (11%) (Table 7.3). Only 1–5% of all breast cancers present as nipple discharge. Ductal adenomas more commonly present as a breast mass but may occasionally present as bloody nipple discharge. When a pathologic nipple discharge was associated with a palpable mass, there was a greater likelihood of identifying a carcinoma at the time of biopsy.

EVALUATION AND TREATMENT OF NIPPLE DISCHARGE

When the patient presents to the office with the complaint of nipple discharge, the first step is a careful history to determine into which category the discharge falls, galactorrhea, physiologic or pathologic. If the history is suggestive of galactorrhea, a careful menstrual history and drug history should be obtained. There are many medications which are associated with galactorrhea and most can be safely stopped or changed. In addition, the patient should be questioned about symptoms related to thyroid dysfunction and visual field deficits to rule out thyroid disease and a pituitary adenoma, respectively.

When the diagnosis of galactorrhea is being considered, a prolactin level and thyroid function tests should be obtained. If an abnormality in thyroid function is found, it should be evaluated and treated. When persistent hyperprolactinemia is identified, the patient should undergo evaluation for a pituitary adenoma by computed tomography or magnetic resonance imaging. If a pituitary tumor is identified the patient should be referred for neurosurgical evaluation. Individuals with advanced pituitary tumors may have visual field deficits which may be identified by visual field testing. Patients with moderately elevated prolactin levels without radiologic evidence of a pituitary adenoma should be followed closely. Transient elevation of prolactin levels has been associated with breast stimulation, chest trauma or thoracotomy. Patients with idiopathic galactorrhea which is severe and regular menses may be treated effectively with ergot derivatives as a means to reduce the prolactin level. Bromocriptine has been utilized to treat patients with idiopathic galactorrhea associated with amenorrhea. Galactorrhea should not be treated with a surgical duct excision. Often, physiologic discharge can be distinguished from pathologic discharge by history, since physiologic discharge is generally bilateral and not spontaneous whereas pathologic discharge is unilateral and spontaneous.

No matter what the cause of the discharge, a thorough breast examination should be performed and other physical findings such as retraction or eczema of the nipple, dimpling of the skin, inflammatory changes, a breast mass and axillary adenopathy should be excluded. In addition, the quadrant of the breast where compression results in fluid production should be identified and if fluid is obtained, it should be tested for occult blood. In cases of galactorrhea or physiologic nipple discharge where the fluid is guaiac negative, the patient should be reassured that there is no serious underlying breast pathology when the breast examination is negative. Mammography is recommended if it is appropriate for the patient's age and she has not had one performed within the year.

Patients who present with a pathologic nipple discharge should have a mammogram as part of the initial evaluation. A radiographic finding may shed light on the underlying condition such as (1) mammary duct ectasia which may be manifested as a dilated duct and (2) a carcinoma which may be manifested by either a mass or microcalcifications. A negative mammogram does not preclude an occult carcinoma, as Tabar reported that only half of the patients in his study who presented with nipple discharge and were diagnosed with breast cancer had an abnormal mammogram.

There have been no definite benefits identified for the routine use of cytology in the evaluation of nipple discharge. Numerous authors have reported that carcinomas which present as spontaneous nipple discharge are not routinely identified by cytology. Ciatto and colleagues found that only 14 of 31 patients with breast cancer presenting as nipple discharge had suspicious cytology. An additional eight patients with suspicious cytology had either papillomas or some other benign diagnosis after surgical duct excision. Therefore, the decision to proceed with a terminal duct excision for pathologic nipple discharge should not be based upon cytology but rather upon other clinical factors. Cytology in the postpartum patient with bloody nipple discharge commonly leads to false-positive interpretations, and therefore is not recommended.

Galactography was introduced over 60 years ago but was not widely utilized until the 1960s. It has been utilized in evaluating patients with pathologic nipple discharge to identify intraductal pathology and is relatively easy to perform;

however, its routine use in this clinical setting is controversial. Tabar suggests that all patients who present with either bloody or serous nipple discharge from a single duct should undergo galactography and some authors have suggested that surgery may be avoided when the galactogram is negative. It is not recommended in women with mastitis or breast abscess, since it may exacerbate the inflammatory process.

The procedure entails the identification and cannulation of the secreting duct, followed by injection of a sterile water-soluble contrast material. Compression of the quadrant of the breast producing the fluid can aid in the identification of the secreting orifice. The process of cannulating the duct is often the most difficult portion of the procedure and may be facilitated by good lighting and either using a magnifying glass or a dissecting microscope. A plastic catheter or a blunt sialography needle can be used to cannulate the duct. After injection of the contrast, mammography is then performed and films are taken in two views. Some have advocated injecting the abnormal duct with a dilute methylene blue solution just prior to the excision so that it can be performed more precisely and result in less breast tissue being removed.

Galactography may be able to define ductal anatomy and identify intraductal lesions; however, it does not distinguish between benign versus malignant intraductal lesions and is not routinely recommended. It may play a role in identifying lesions which are located peripherally in the ductal system or in women with large breasts where a lesion might not be resected during the course of the routine duct excision (Table 7.4).

Fiberoptic ductoscopy has been recently introduced as a means to evaluate patients with spontaneous nipple discharge and may prove to be useful in identifying intraductal lesions.

TECHNIQUES OF TERMINAL DUCT EXCISION

At the time of surgery, if preoperative galactography was not performed and methylene

Table 7.4 Evaluation of pathologic nipple discharge

- History and physical examination
- Occult blood
- Mammogram
- Galactography

blue dye was not injected into the duct, the secreting duct can be cannulated with a lacrimal duct probe to aid in the dissection and in limiting the resection of breast tissue. A circumareolar incision which encompasses approximately half of the circumference of the areola is most commonly used. The incision should be placed to gain the greatest exposure, as the quadrant of the breast from where the discharge is from should be known. Others have advocated the use of a radial incision extending across the areola to the nipple. The full thickness of the areola is elevated sharply as a flap to gain exposure to the terminal ducts. Meticulous hemostasis should be obtained. At this point, if one identifies a single, dilated duct, it is then excised. If multiple ducts are dilated or if none appear grossly abnormal, the entire main ductal system is excised. In each case, the dissection is carried back away from the nipple for a distance of approximately 3–5 cm and a cone of tissue is excised. The specimen is transected at the dermis of the nipple to ensure that superficial intraductal lesions will be removed. Deep tissues are not reapproximated and drains are not placed, since this may lead to a subsequent cosmetic deformity. Interrupted absorbable sutures are used to bring the areola back into its normal position and the skin is then closed with a running subcuticular suture.

Complications after terminal duct excision are uncommon. It is rare that a patient would experience reduced sensation of the nipple or necrosis of the nipple–areolar complex. Patients who undergo terminal duct excision for duct ectasia or periareolar sepsis may develop recurrent infections requiring additional surgery. Women of childbearing years should be advised that breastfeeding after a terminal duct excision is not possible. However, a selective duct excision where only the secreting duct is excised can be performed in a woman who requires a duct excision and wishes to maintain her ability to breastfeed.

Bibliography

Barnes AB. Medical intelligence current concepts. Diagnosis and treatment of abnormal breast secretions. *N Engl J Med* 1966;275:1184–7

Ciatto S, Bravetti P, Cariaggi P. Significance of nipple discharge. Clinical patterns in the selection of patients for cytologic examination. *Acta Cytol* 1986; 30:17–20

Chaudary MA, Millis RR, Davies GC, *et al.* Nipple discharge. *Ann Surg* 1982;196:651–5

Funderburk WW, Syphax B. Evaluation of nipple discharge in benign and malignant diseases. *Cancer* 1969;24:1290–6

Kleinberg D, Noel G, Frantz A. Galactorrhea: a study of 235 cases, including 48 with pituitary tumors. *N Engl J Med* 1977;296:589–600

Kline TS, Lash SR. Bleeding nipple of pregnancy and postpartum period: cytologic and histologic study. *Acta Cytol* 1964;8:336–40

Lafreniere R. Bloody nipple discharge during pregnancy: a rationale for conservative treatment. *J Surg Oncol* 1990;43:228–30

Morrow M. In: Harris JR, Hellman S, Henderson IC, *et al.*, eds. *Nipple Discharge*. Philadelphia: JB Lippincott, 1987:72–7

Tabar L, Dean PB, Pentek Z. Galactography. *Radiology* 1983;149:31–8

Urban J. Excision of the major duct system of the breast. *Cancer* 1963;16:516–20

Infectious disorders of the breast

8

B.A. Eskin

Most disturbing of the benign processes that affect the breast tissues are those that result from infection and its sequelae. Nipple infections commonly occur during nursing but are easily correctable. They may require only short-term limitations on breastfeedings with the affected breast. However, puerperal (pregnant and post-partum) and non-puerperal breast infections are fraught with serious complications. Particular emphasis must be placed on the relevant symptoms and signs and immediate therapy started. Otherwise undesirable consequences in function, stability and cosmetic results follow. Recent studies have shown that in multiparous women with a previous infectious mastitis, the probability of infection in a subsequent puerperium is threefold.

PUERPERAL MASTITIS

Puerperal or lactational mastitis is an acute cellulitis of the lactating breast that, if untreated, progresses to abscess formation. Puerperal mastitis may occur in both epidemic and sporadic forms.

Sporadic puerperal mastitis presents as cellulitis in a wedge-shaped pattern over a portion of breast skin. Often there is a cracked or irritated nipple, evidently the point of entry for bacteria. Episodes of mastitis occur most commonly during the early weeks of nursing, when nipple trauma is most frequent. The nipple area has not become accustomed to suckling, as yet. The affected wedge of breast tissue is red, warm, and exquisitely tender. The infection is around, rather than within, the ductal system and generally there is no purulent drainage from the nipple, although an increased number of white blood cells (WBC) may be observed in the milk. Fevers to 39 or 40°C with chills and flu-like aching are common.

Diagnosis and treatment

In its early stages, sporadic puerperal mastitis must be distinguished from milk stasis, resulting from duct obstruction and from non-infectious inflammation of the breast. With duct obstruction, there is tenderness and engorgement of the involved breast segment, but no fever or erythema. Normal milk, obtained in the absence of inflammatory symptoms, contains fewer than 10^6 WBC/ml and fewer than 10^3 bacteria/ml. With plugged ducts and milk stasis, in the absence of infection, these normal values are maintained. With non-infectious inflammation, WBC counts may rise to more than 10^6/ml, but milk remains sterile or shows fewer than 10^3 bacteria/ml. In infectious mastitis, however, there are more than 10^6 WBC/ml and bacterial counts exceed 10^3/ml.

Antibiotics should be started in cases with elevation of both WBC and bacterial counts, and clinical judgment is required when only one infectious element is seen. If antibiotic treatment is initiated before the stage of suppuration and abscess formation, there can be complete resolution of puerperal mastitis.

The most commonly isolated organism in puerperal mastitis is *Staphylococcus aureus*; hence, empiric antibiotic therapy should cover this pathogen. While it is not clear whether the infectious organism comes from the mother's skin or the infant's mouth, research data suggest the former. All episodes of early mastitis respond promptly to antibiotic therapy with penicillin, dicloxacillin, or erythromycin. Interestingly, penicillin therapy was effective even in women whose cultured *S. aureus* was penicillin-resistant. Thus, culture and sensitivity results are not predictive of clinical outcome and are probably not necessary if the puerperal mastitis is treated early. The presence of sero–sanguinous fluid or thick yellow discharge from the nipple requires prompt action (see breast abscesses, below).

Historically, puerperal mastitis was treated with prompt weaning, binding of the breasts, and agents, usually hormonal, to stop lactation. It has become clear, however, that these measures increase milk stasis and breast engorgement and, in fact, may contribute to abscess formation. This concept is supported by the finding that many episodes of mastitis follow periods of missed feedings or attempts at weaning, both situations that may result in prolonged breast engorgement. A woman with puerperal mastitis is now encouraged to breastfeed or pump the affected breast to promote drainage of milk from the involved segments. This process also increases vascularity to the affected segment. Warmth and manual pressure to involved areas may also decrease engorgement and speed resolution. The suckling infant is not adversely affected by nursing from an affected breast and does not require antibiotics.

Epidemic puerperal mastitis, or acute mammary adenitis, occurs in hospital maternity wards and can usually be traced to a carrier of the infectious bacteria. The nursing infant harbors the pathogen orally, acquiring it from the carrier or from contact with the mother's skin. The sequence of infection is believed to be initiated by heavy contamination through an active nipple by the pathogen. Regurgitation by the infant forces the bacteria into multiple lactiferous ducts at the nipple. Heavy seeding into multiple ducts is assumed, since the infection appears simultaneously in several of the non-adjacent segments of the breast. These segments are red, warm, and tender, but not fluctuant. *S. aureus* is the most common organism implicated in puerperal mastitis, regardless of etiology. Since the infant harbors the pathogen, weaning is necessary to prevent recurrent infection. Antibiotic administration is indicated with warmth, manual pressure, and pumping to the affected breast, which is the same treatment as was used in sporadic puerperal mastitis. Fortunately, epidemic puerperal mastitis has become infrequent, probably because of improved hygiene and shorter hospital stays postpartum.

BREAST ABSCESSES

Puerperal

If puerperal mastitis is not treated quickly enough or fails to respond to conservative measures, an abscess may form. Once an abscess is perceived, incision and draining become mandatory. Fluctuance may be often absent or difficult to detect when numerous fibrous septa are present within the breast. The rule of thumb is that when tenderness and erythema of puerperal mastitis remain after antibiotic therapy, the presence of an abscess should be assumed, and incision and drainage should be performed. An anesthetic is usually desirable and since local infection with local anesthesia would be hazardous, a general anesthetic may be required for the procedure. Abscesses are usually single, peripherally located, and contain multiple loculations. A linear incision is made over the area of maximum tenderness at the point of the abscess. The skin is retracted and all loculations are broken up to ensure resolution of the abscess. In rare neglected cases, the abscess can extend below the pectoralis major fascia, which then requires adequate drainage. A biopsy of the abscess wall is recommended by a few authors to rule out previously unrecognized coexisting carcinoma.

Traditionally, after incision and drainage, the abscess is either packed open or loosely closed over a drain brought out through a separate dependent incision. The drain can be brought out through the same initial incision depending on the size of the drain needed and the length of time it will remain in place.

There are now several advocates for tissue curettage of the abscess cavity with primary closure, appropriate antibiotic coverage, and no drain, if shallow. In sharp contrast to subareolar, non-puerperal breast abscesses, healing of puerperal abscesses is generally prompt, and development of fistulae is rare, regardless of the form of drainage employed. Although some authors have stated that antibiotic coverage is unnecessary after proper drainage of a puerperal breast abscess, most clinicians currently favor a brief course of antibiotics after drainage.

Non-puerperal

Several large hospitals have reported that only 8.5% of breast abscesses seen over a 10-year period were puerperal abscesses. Surprisingly, non-lactational breast abscesses constitute most breast abscesses seen in clinical practice. These breast abscesses are mostly subareolar, and have an indolent and relapsing course. A fraction of non-lactating patients will present with acute peripheral abscesses which are similar to puerperal mastitis. Subareolar abscesses do not cause systemic illnesses in most cases. There is an area of tenderness, erythema, and induration under periareolar skin.

Often, the abscess remains peripheral to the areola when treated with simple incision and drainage. Complications and recurrence may result in 50% of patients. This high percentage is due to other conditions that predispose to infections, such as diabetes, steroid therapy, or other infected skin lesions, not usually seen in patients with subareolar abscesses.

Organisms cultured from non-puerperal breast abscesses differ from those cultured from puerperal abscesses. *Staphylococcus aureus* is the most common organism found in puerperal abscesses and is usually solitary. In contrast, non-puerperal abscesses usually yield multiple organisms, including anaerobes. The apocrine apparatus in the subareolar tissue creates an environment favoring the growth of anaerobic and mixed infections. For that reason, empirical antibiotic coverage should be broad spectrum and include good coverage for anaerobic organisms.

The range of cultures found has been markedly variable. In a series from 47 non-puerperal breast abscesses, 87% yielded 2.2 species of organisms per specimen. Thirty-four of 41 specimens grew anaerobes, usually *Bacteroides*, while the remaining seven specimens grew pure cultures of *S. aureus*. In another series, bacteria from non-puerperal breast abscesses averaged 3.6 bacterial species per isolate. Eighty-six per cent of samples grew anaerobes with mostly *Peptostreptococcus* and *Proprionibacterium*. Coagulase-negative *Staphylococcus* species were the most common aerobes, while only three samples (88%) grew *S. aureus*.

Etiology

Many factors contribute to the appearance of non-puerperal breast abscesses. Abscesses clearly may be part of the syndrome of duct ectasia (Chapter 9), arising either as part of the process of periductal mastitis or by secondary infection of dilated, secretion-filled ducts. Nipple inversion is one of the etiologic factors which predispose to formation of subareolar breast abscesses. The abscess communicates with a duct which lies in the interspace created by inversion of the nipple. Chronic inflammation of tissues around an inverted nipple may lead to bacterial colonization with abscess formation. Some authors suggest that the nipple inversion is secondary to scarring produced by the chronic inflammation, rather than being a primary factor contributing to the initial infection. A relatively low percentage of abscesses with nipple inversion suggest that it is not essential for secondary abscess formation.

Treatment

Antibiotic treatment and/or simple incision and drainage (I&D) is inadequate therapy for most non-puerperal breast abscesses, particularly those in a subareolar or periareolar location. The occasional peripherally located abscess which appears in a non-lactational setting and shows active *S. aureus* is effectively treated by incision and drainage and appropriate antibiotic coverage. Recurrence of these abscesses is uncommon. An occasional infected sebaceous cyst may appear in breast tissue and should be treated with warm soaks, interim I&D, and excision of the cyst wall following subsidence of the acute inflammation and edema.

The common non-puerperal breast abscess, which is found subareolarly, has a high recurrence rate after standard I&D, and antibiotic therapy does not decrease this recidivism. It is believed that the underlying pathologies (i.e., damaged ducts with obstruction and surrounding accumulated debris) remain after I&D, leading to a recurrence of the infection and abscess within 2–3 weeks.

The Hadfield procedure, the consensus opinion, which requires incision and drainage of the abscesses, should be done in the acute phase, followed by broad-spectrum antibiotics. Many authors believe that a biopsy from the wall of the abscess cavity should be taken and this tissue examined to rule out coexisting carcinoma. Following the resolution of the acute inflammatory process, the major ducts beneath the areola are excised through a circumareolar skin incision. This may further require a periareolar abscess drainage site when significant induration continues to be present. The core of tissue excised often includes the terminal ducts beneath the nipple with their first divisions. In the Hadfield procedure, the tissues remaining after duct excision and the skin are opposed by primary closure, which has the advantage of minimal cosmetic deformity. Most patients will heal without a recurrence of the abscess.

Simple mastectomy has occasionally been required for recurrent subareolar abscesses. In light of current knowledge concerning etiology and physiology, radical treatment is rarely necessary.

PREGNANCY, NURSING, AND DUCT INCISIONS

Women who have a pregnancy following major duct excisions carry their pregnancies to term without any breast problems. The general policy has been to discourage patients from attempting to breastfeed after any deep procedures. Lactation occurs naturally in the non-operated breast, but milk is not discharged from the operated side. During the first year after major duct excision, there is some engorgement of the operated breast during pregnancy. With cessation of breastfeeding, this enlargement subsides sooner than the non-operated side. After several years, pregnancy results in only minimal engorgement in the operated breast which suggests that atrophy of acinar tissue has occurred secondary to duct resection.

MAMMARY FISTULAE

In the past, fistulae were a common complication of incision and drainage of puerperal breast abscesses. Fistulae have become complications of duct ectasias, but remain uncommon. Long-standing subareolar breast abscesses may progress to form a fistulous tract by epithelialization of the drainage tract. In these cases, the fistula originates from a dilated subareolar duct and usually empties through an opening in the periareolar skin. A probe placed into the fistulous tract will pass through this duct and exit through the nipple.

Fistulae may arise after breast biopsies and surgical or spontaneous drainage of subareolar abscesses. An important and common cause is the high incidence of inverted nipples. There has been discussion as to whether nipple inversion is causative or secondary to inflammation and scarring, resulting in fistulae. Organisms recovered from mammary duct fistulae and in non-puerperal breast abscesses are similar.

Fistulae are treated by first opening them over a probe. The tract is excised with the involved duct and the specific portion of the nipple through which the involved duct passed. Leaving any segment of the involved duct within the nipple predisposes to recurrence. The surgical wound is packed open and allowed to granulate in. Healing requires 4–6 weeks, but final cosmetic results are quite good and recurrence is uncommon.

UNCOMMON INFLAMMATORY LESIONS

Rare causes of mammary duct fistulae and abscesses include tuberculosis, syphilis, and fungal infections. These unusual infections are diagnosed by the appropriate stains, cultures, and serologic tests.

Granulomatous lobular mastitis has been seen to produce inflammatory masses in the breast. Granulomatous inflammation of the lobules when seen on histopathology may produce extensive necrosis. This lesion is more common in younger women, sometimes occurring during pregnancy, puerperium, or lactation. No infectious agent has been identified, and there is no apparent association with trauma, breast-feeding, or oral contraceptive use. This condition is generally treated with steroids and has a chronic and relapsing course. Surgical resection of involved areas is reserved for intractable cases.

Neonatal mastitis, seen as swelling of sub-areolar tissue in a newborn, is not an infectious process (Chapter 2). The swelling that occurs is considered to be in response to transplacental passage of maternal hormones, particularly estrogen, and disappears soon after birth.

Bibliography

Aitken RJ, Hood J, Going JJ, *et al.* Bacteriology of mammary duct ectasia. *Br J Surg* 1988;75:1040–1

Benson EA. Management of breast abscesses. *World J Surg* 1989;13:753–6

Brook I. Microbiology of non-puerperal breast abscesses. *J Infect Dis* 1988;157:377–9

Bundred NJ, Dixon JM, Chetty U, *et al.* Mammillary fistula. *Br J Surg* 1987;74:466–8

Bundred NJ, Dixon JMJ, Lumsden AB, *et al.* Are the lesions of duct ectasia sterile? *Br J Surg* 1985;72:844–5

Dixon JM, Chetty U, Forrest APM. Wound infection after breast biopsy. *Br J Surg* 1988;75:918–19

Dixon JM. Periductal mastitis/duct ectasia. *World J Surg* 1989;13:715–20

Going JJ, Anderson TJ, Wilkinson S, *et al.* Granulomatous lobular mastitis. *J Clin Pathol* 1987;40:535–40

Hadfield GH. Further experience of the operation for the excision of the major duct system of the breast. *Br J Surg* 1968;55:530–5

Walker AP, Edmiston CE, Krepel CJ, *et al.* A prospective study of the microflora of nonpuerperal breast abscess. *Arch Surg* 1988;12:908–11

Mammary duct ectasia

9

L. Jardines

INTRODUCTION

This condition is also known by a variety of other names such as plasma cell mastitis, mastitis obliterans, comedomastitis, periductal mastitis and secretory disease of the breast. This disease process occurs primarily in women but has been reported in men as well. The pathogenesis of mammary duct ectasia is not understood well and different theories have been proposed. The most recent suggests that periductal inflammation leads to destruction of the elastic lamina of the duct resulting in dilatation. This theory fits with the observation that young patients with this condition have a picture of periductal inflammation and older patients tend to have ductal dilatation as the primary histologic finding.

Histologically, one sees dilated terminal ducts of the breast which can be filled with stagnant secretions and keratin. There is an associated inflammatory process composed primarily of plasma cells which surrounds the ducts. Patients with mammary duct ectasia often have nipple secretions which contain bacteria; however, it is not clear whether these bacteria play a role in the pathogenesis of duct ectasia. Patients who undergo a surgical breast biopsy for mammary duct ectasia have a wound infection rate of approximately 10% which is significantly higher than that seen after breast biopsy for other reasons.

INCIDENCE

The exact incidence of mammary duct ectasia in the population is not known, since there are many women with this disorder who are asymptomatic. Mammary duct ectasia is the underlying cause of symptoms in 1–2% of women referred to a breast clinic. In patients who presented with breast complaints and underwent biopsy, mammary duct ectasia was identified in 4.2%. Approximately 8% of patients who underwent breast surgery for other reasons were found to have mammary duct ectasia as an incidental finding. In some reports, where breast tissue was studied in post-mortem examination, the incidence of mammary duct ectasia was as high as 24%.

PRESENTATION

The age at presentation with symptomatic mammary duct ectasia ranges from <30 to >80 years, with the peak incidence seen in the 40–49 year age group. Mammary duct ectasia can present in a variety of ways, including nipple discharge, a breast mass, breast abscess, nipple retraction, mammary fistula and/or breast pain (Table 9.1).

A breast mass secondary to mammary duct ectasia is most commonly seen in the region of

Table 9.1 Presentation of mammary duct ectasia

- Nipple discharge
- Breast mass
- Breast abscess, generally retroareolar
- Nipple retraction
- Mammary fistula
- Breast pain

the areola, but can also be seen peripherally within the breast. This diagnosis accounts for approximately 3–4% of all benign breast masses overall but is seen in a greater percentage of biopsies performed in women over the age of 55. In older women, it may be difficult to distinguish a mass secondary to mammary duct ectasia from one related to an underlying carcinoma. In both instances, the mass may be hard, irregular and/or fixed to the surrounding tissues. In addition, there may also be skin or nipple retraction. In most instances, a biopsy of the mass is recommended to establish the diagnosis.

Pain is commonly associated with symptomatic mammary duct ectasia and is generally subareolar. It is more likely to be seen in younger patients with mammary duct ectasia. The pain may be either cyclical or non-cyclical. It has been suggested that antibiotics directed against the common organisms seen in mammary duct ectasia may be useful in treating the pain, since it may be related to the periductal inflammation.

Nipple discharge is seen in approximately 15–20% of patients with mammary duct ectasia. The discharge may be unilateral or bilateral and fluid may be produced from a single duct or multiple ducts. Fluid production may be spontaneous or may result only with breast compression or stimulation. The color of the fluid varies from clear, green, yellow, creamy, brown and (less likely) bloody (either grossly or occult). When the fluid production is bilateral and multiple ducts are involved, the likelihood of an underlying malignancy is remote. Nipple discharge which is unilateral, from a single duct, spontaneous and persistent, no matter what the color, is considered pathologic and surgery is recommended. Approximately 17–36% of women who present with a pathologic nipple discharge and undergo a terminal duct excision are found to have mammary duct ectasia as the etiology of the discharge.

In 32% of women who undergo breast surgery and are found to have mammary duct ectasia, nipple retraction is the major clinical finding. The age range of the patients presenting with nipple retraction secondary to mammary duct ectasia extends from 25 to 75 years, with a median age of 52 years. The duration of symptoms varies and ranges from 3 months to several years. In 15% of patients, the nipple retraction is bilateral. Nipple inversion secondary to mammary duct ectasia must be distinguished from an underlying breast carcinoma. Retraction from a breast carcinoma is more likely to be complete and associated with distortion of the areola, although these clinical findings cannot reliably distinguish one from the other. Retraction which has been present for over 1 year without an associated mass, and bilateral nipple retraction, are most often associated with a benign etiology. Patients presenting with nipple retraction should undergo a thorough breast examination and mammography. The mammogram may reveal dilated ducts in the retroareolar region or smooth coarse calcifications. Occasionally, the calcifications are periductal and are related to fat necrosis. It has been suggested that patients who have no other finding on breast examination other than nipple retraction and a negative mammogram may be followed closely. If there is an associated breast mass, fine needle aspiration cytology should be considered prior to proceeding with an open surgical biopsy.

Non-puerperal breast abscesses are seen more frequently than abscesses associated with lactation, and when in the periareolar position they are often associated with mammary duct ectasia. A periareolar breast abscess is the presenting problem in less than 10% of patients with symptomatic mammary duct ectasia. As with abscesses in other locations, they often present as a tender, fluctuant mass with overlying erythema with or without signs of systemic sepsis. The patient will often require operative incision and drainage of the abscess in association with antibiotics. The bacteria encountered in breast abscesses secondary to mammary duct ectasia include *Staphylococcus aureus* and anaerobes, particularly *Bacteroides* (Table 9.2). Therefore, antibiotic coverage should be broad

Table 9.2 Bacteriology of abscesses associated with mammary duct ectasia

- *Staphylococcus aureus*
- *Bacteroides*
- Streptococci (aerobic and anaerobic)
- Enterococci

spectrum and provide anaerobic coverage. At the time of surgery, the abscess cavity should be biopsied to rule out an underlying carcinoma. In some instances, the patient may require general anesthesia for the procedure, since these abscesses are generally loculated; however, it is possible to perform the abscess drainage using local anesthesia and intravenous sedation. There is seldom a role for performing incision and drainage of a breast abscess in the emergency department, since it is extremely difficult to provide adequate anesthesia when only local anesthesia is used. When the wound is healed and the inflammatory process has subsided, the patient may require a terminal duct excision to prevent recurrent breast sepsis. Non-puerperal breast abscesses are more likely to recur when they are located in the subareolar position, when anaerobic bacteria are cultured from the wound and when there is underlying mammary duct ectasia. It has also been noted that patients who develop a non-lactational breast abscess and smoke cigarettes are more likely to develop recurrent breast abscesses and mammary fistulae. Those patients who require a terminal duct excision for the treatment of recurrent subareolar sepsis for presumed mammary duct ectasia should be advised that they will be unable to lactate from the operated breast following surgery.

An alternative to operative incision and drainage in the treatment of a breast abscess is aspiration of the purulent material with a large bore needle and administration of broad spectrum antibiotics. The patient may require more than one aspiration of the abscess to control the inflammatory process. The advantage to this method of treatment is that the patient does not require surgery and there is no surgical scar or deformity. This treatment modality should be utilized in patients who are of low risk for breast cancer. Anyone treated in this manner must be followed closely to ensure resolution of the infection and that the abscess is not associated with an underlying malignancy.

The development of a mammary fistula, Zuska's disease, is uncommon, and presents as a draining fistula at the areolar border from the subareolar tissue with or without nipple retraction. The majority of patients who develop a mammary fistula have histologic evidence of mammary duct ectasia. It is seen most frequently in patients who have undergone incision and drainage of a breast abscess but is also seen after breast biopsy without septic complications. Different treatment regimens have been described; however, it is probably necessary to excise the fistula and the affected ducts to prevent recurrence. The use of perioperative antibiotics may also reduce the likelihood of developing a recurrent fistula.

Bibliography

Asch T, Frey C. Radiographic appearance of mammary-duct ectasia with calcification. *N Engl J Med* 1962;266: 86–7

Browning J, Briggs A, Taylor I. Symptomatic and incidental mammary duct ectasia. *Br J Med* 1986;79:715–16

Bundred NJ, Dixon JM, Forrest APM. Mammillary fistula. *Br J Surg* 1987;74:466–8

Bundred NJ, Dover MS, Coley S, *et al*. Breast abscesses and cigarette smoking. *Br J Surg* 1992;79: 58–9

Dixon JM. Periductal mastitis/duct ectasia. *World J Surg* 1989;13:715–20

Dixon JM, Anderson TJ, Lumsden AB, *et al*. Mammary duct ectasia. *Br J Surg* 1983;70:601–3

Rees BI, Gravelle IH, Hughes LE. Nipple retraction in duct ectasia. *Br J Surg* 1977;64:577–80

Scholefield JH, Duncan JL, Rogers K. Review of a hospital experience of breast abscesses. *Br J Surg* 1987;74:469–70

Webb AJ. Mammary duct ectasia–periductal mastitis complex. *Br J Surg* 1995;82:1300–2

Fibrocystic disease of the breast 10

B.A. Eskin

INTRODUCTION

The most common benign diseases of the breast seen in the premenopausal woman fall into a catch-all category defined as *fibrocystic disease*. The major pathognomonic findings are benign fluid retention (cysts) that occurs in the ducts and the accompanying periductal fibrosis. This results often from inflammatory or traumatic conditions, notably in the connective tissues. Symptoms consist of lumpy and enlarged breasts with the most severe discomfort generally premenstrually.

Breast diseases, in general, appear to be age-dependent, peaking during the deceleration period of reproduction. After menopause, benign breast disease diminishes and malignancy increases proportionately. A significant increase in incidence of breast cancer has been shown with each 5-year increment in age, an observation which is particularly convincing in menopause. Benign disease is less likely when masses are palpated in the breasts of post-menopausal women. This reflects the importance of the reproductive cyclic changes that occur in premenopausal women as a probable etiology for that benign change. Duct and gland prominence decreases and results in diminished nodularities with age.

Reclassification of fibrocystic diseases was recommended by the American College of Pathology in order to provide better characterizations of the specific components of benign specimens obtained at biopsy. This would allow for better interpretation for determining which fibrocystic tissues may be precancerous. Descriptions include cystic morphology, stromal cellular variations and glandular hypertrophy and hyperplasia.

Breasts are significantly easier to examine both by palpation and radiographically than internal organs. However, radiologists who read mammograms are confounded by the distortions seen when fibrocystic disease is marked. Needle aspiration of the cysts with histopathology of the fluid obtained often helps radiologic diagnosis. Biopsy is recommended whenever diagnosis by mammogram and palpation of the lesion continues to waver between benign and malignant.

With menopause, estrogen and progesterone stimuli are reduced, with an evident decrease in fibrocystic disease caused by a declining steroid activity. The accepted use of estrogen replacement therapy has been seen to result in recurrences in some cases in those women who had evident premenopausal fibrocystic disease. The estrogen serum levels obtained in women given estrogen replacement therapy are less than those seen during the reproductive years, so that this problem is not prevalent.

DIAGNOSIS OF BREAST DISEASE

The general purpose of the various breast diagnostic techniques described elsewhere is to differentiate benign from malignant diseases. Benign breast changes generally parallel sex hormone release each reproductive month. These functional variants begin at menarche (onset of bleeding) and plateau during the transitional or premenopausal period. Examination of the breasts should be done immediately after menses, when steroid hormone levels are lowest. During the premenopause when cycle lengths vary, often examinations provide erroneous results. After menopause, a minimal amount of intrinsic estrogen will still be present. This is always less than that required to bring about significant changes in the breast tissue and to provide a menses.

Techniques commonly used for breast diagnosis are physical examination (palpation) (Chapter 4), mammography and ultrasound (Chapter 5), and histopathologic evaluation by needle biopsy or tissue biopsy (Chapter 11). Ancillary evaluations by aspiration of cystic structures and nipple excretion testing with cytology are often required (Chapter 7). Other methods which are in use are: diaphanography, thermography (often color coded), and chemical determinations by computer densitometry.

Early detection of breast cancer lesions that are 1 cm or less is predictive of a longer survival for the woman. Thus, a careful and systematic evaluation is advised. In young women, self breast examination (SBE) is taught by physicians and nurses, so that suspicious lumps can be reported to the primary physician for further characterization. While meeting with controversy, the technique of SBE remains useful to those women who are willing to follow the program carefully and report immediately any discrepancy in their breast contour. Because of the density of the breasts, postmenopausal self examination is physically more difficult and less accurate. Physician routine breast examinations should be done every 6 months, or at least yearly. Physician techniques are described and demonstrated in Chapter 4.

The American Cancer Society made recommendations that mammography be done routinely: (a) once as a baseline before 40 years; (b) every 18–24 months in the forties; (c) yearly in the fifties; and (d) thereafter as indicated. Several media-generated modifications in this training have been published, causing confusion to the women in the critical populations. Recently, evidence that women in their forties may increase the interims (greater than 2 years) between mammographies has been refuted, particularly in those with breast risk factors. Physicians and scientists at a summary program at the National Cancer Institute in Washington, DC, in 1997 further confounded the issue. They returned the 40–50-year-old woman to a variable time-frame determined by unstated risk, symptoms and availability. Individuals who are at risk would require mammography more often. However, the Radiologic Society of America feels that the dangers from the radiation given from low-dose mammography presents a much lower risk than the potential of breast cancer, and continues the previous recommendations. Chapter 5 describes some of the proposed modifications.

Fibrocystic disease is important diagnostically. It often distorts physical examination, palpations and mammography, causing small lesions to be missed. When a cyst is easily palpated, needle aspiration using ultrasound localization often helps. Fibrocystic disease in menopausal women tends to be minimal, firmer, and with reduced cystic changes. When the lumps are suspicious by palpation or as a radiologic density, tissue biopsy is appropriate. Some surgeons feel that needle biopsy is sufficiently accurate and less invasive if the lesion is accessible.

Physician palpation and breast self-examination can feel a distinct mass only when greater than 1 cm. Growth pattern studies report that when a lesion is palpable at 1 cm, it has been growing for 8 years. Newer radiographic techniques detect breast cancer lesions approximately 3 years before they are palpated. Therefore, mammography screening may reduce mortality as much as 30%. The downside of routine mammographies is cost, discomfort, radiation exposure and inconvenience for the patients. Using the newer methods and X-ray units, the average radiation dose to the sternum is 50 mrad and this hazard decreases after the age of 35. Most physicians will avoid use of radiologic techniques in young women, if possible, by using ultrasound, diaphanography, and in some cases magnetic resonance.

Office diagnostic techniques

Several office techniques are available which may provide an early, apparently accurate diagnosis. Primary physicians, when qualified, are justified to follow up the presence of a palpable or mammographic lesion. A mass is considered dominant when it is palpable in two dimensions.

Office ultrasound and diaphanography help differentiate the consistency of lumps and provide some indication of fluid or solid content. Aspiration of the lesion is recommended whenever fluid is believed to be present and is attainable. Cytologic examination of the aspirate from these masses is investigated fully when it is thickened, bloody or discolored; otherwise, the aspirate is discarded. Should more tissue remain within the site after this procedure, further localization using ultrasound or X-ray with tissue biopsy must be done.

The value of fine needle aspiration of the breast remains controversial and dependent on the skill of the physician. The false-negative rate for needle aspiration remains uncomfortably variable because of this (5–40%). Pathologists state that cancer cells do not adhere well to the aspirating needle, so that the major flaw in the procedure is that the neoplastic cells, if present, are not always obtained. Several major centers use this technique because positive results are usually correct (3.2% false-positive) and immediate positive reports reduce delay in therapy. Methods for this test are amply described in Chapter 10.

Invasive diagnostic techniques in the office are usually done only by breast surgeons, since they have final responsibility for excision and therapeutic support, should cancer be present. Whether a positive frozen section or surgical biopsy should indicate the need to advance immediately to an invasive radical procedure remains controversial.

When a mass seen by mammography, ultrasound, or diaphanography cannot be palpated, the level of suspicion requires evaluation with a full knowledge of risk and history. If the lesion is questionable, an immediate needle localization biopsy is required. Survival potential can be increased by immediate action and reducing the chance of metastasis.

BENIGN DISEASES

The term *benign breast disorders* encompasses a heterogeneous group of lesions that clinically and radiographically span the entire spectrum of breast abnormalities. Those that present as localized masses must be distinguished from carcinoma. When that priority is met, pathologic categorization of benign breast lesions will provide useful information on the patient's risk for subsequently developing carcinoma.

In this section, the diagnoses of benign breast problems most commonly reported by the pathologist will be described. Table 10.1 contains a summary of the major histologic categories and how they relate as risks for developing the malignant conditions. Further evaluations of the tissue diagnoses can provide prognostic assistance. However, even using these newer methods, diagnoses still remain evasive in at least 10% of the benign lesions that are proliferative histologically.

Table 10.1 Summary of breast cancer risk related to histologic findings in benign breast biopsies

Histologic category	Relative risk
Non-proliferative	
All patients	0.89
No family history	0.86
Family history*	1.2
Proliferative without atypia	
All patients	1.6
No family history	1.5
Family history*	2.1
Atypical hyperplasia	
All patients	4.4
No family history	3.5
Family history*	8.9

*History of breast cancer in a mother, sister, or daughter.

Fibrocystic disease

Definition

Although the term *fibrocystic disease* is used both by clinicians and pathologists, it does not represent a distinct entity, either clinically or pathologically. This term, along with synonyms such as 'chronic cystic mastitis' and 'mammary dysplasia', is used to describe a heterogeneous group of abnormalities that may occur separately or together.

Clinically, this term has been applied to a condition in which there are palpable breast masses that may fluctuate with the menstrual cycle and are often associated with pain or tenderness. However, at least 60–85% of women have palpably irregular breasts, and in most women these palpable lumps probably represent physiologic changes rather than a pathologic process. Pathologically, the changes included under the heading of fibrocystic disease include macroscopic and microscopic cysts, stromal fibrosis, apocrine metaplasia, and a variety of proliferative lesions.

The majority of patients who have breast biopsies showing fibrocystic disease have non-proliferative lesions and are not at a substantially increased risk of developing breast cancer (Table 10.2). Several multicentered studies have clearly demonstrated that, by separating the various histologic components of fibrocystic disease, subgroups of patients with different risks for subsequently developing carcinoma become apparent.

The system for classifying benign breast lesions, supported at a consensus meeting of the College of American Pathologists, provides a pragmatic, clinically useful approach. This system separates the various components of fibrocystic disease into three groups, with different relative risks for the subsequent development of breast cancer: non-proliferative lesions, proliferative lesions without atypia, and atypical hyperplasias (see Table 10.2).

Non-proliferative lesions These lesions include cysts, papillary apocrine change, epithelial-

Table 10.2 Fibrocystic diseases of the breast

Non-proliferative lesions
 Breast cysts
 Papillary apocrine
 Epithelial-related calcifications
 Mild hyperplasia
 Fibroadenoma
Proliferative lesions without atypia
 Moderate or florid hyperplasia
 Intraductal papillomas
 Sclerosing adenosis
Atypical hyperplasia
 Ductal
 Lobular

related calcifications, mild hyperplasia of the usual type, and fibroadenomas. *Cysts* are fluid-filled, round to ovoid structures that vary in size. *Gross cysts* are those that are large enough to produce palpable masses. Cysts are usually derived from the terminal duct lobular unit, although cystic structures in the more peripheral ducts have been described. The epithelium consists of two layers: an inner (luminal) epithelial layer and an outer myoepithelial layer. In some cysts, the epithelium is markedly attenuated or absent; in others, the lining epithelium shows apocrine metaplasia, characterized by granular eosinophilic cytoplasm and apical cytoplasmic protrusions. *Papillary apocrine change* is characterized by a proliferation of ductal epithelial cells in which all of the cells show apocrine features. *Epithelial-related secondary calcifications* are frequently observed in breast tissue and may be seen in normal ducts and lobules or in virtually any pathologic condition in the breast. It should also be noted that calcifications may also be seen in the breast stroma as well as in blood vessel walls. *Mild hyperplasia of the usual type* is defined as an increase in the number of epithelial cells within a duct that is more than two, but not more than four, epithelial cells in depth. In this type of hyperplasia, the epithelial cells do not cross the lumen of the involved space.

The only patients in the non-proliferative category with an increased risk of developing breast cancer are those with gross cysts plus a family history of breast cancer.

Proliferative lesions without atypia Included within the group of proliferative lesions without atypia are moderate or florid hyperplasias, intraductal papillomas, and sclerosing adenosis. Moderate or florid hyperplasias are intraductal epithelial proliferations that are more than four epithelial cells in depth. They are characterized by a tendency to bridge and often distend the involved space. The proliferation may have a solid, fenestrated, or papillary architecture. If spaces remain within the duct lumen, they are irregular and variable in shape. The cells constituting this type of proliferation are cytologically benign and variable in size, shape, and orientation. It is often possible to discern two distinct cell populations: epithelial cells and myoepithelial cells. A fibrovascular stroma is sometimes present.

Sclerosing adenosis is most often an incidental microscopic finding, but it may present as a palpable mass (adenosis tumor). Microscopically, these lesions consist of a proliferation of acinar structures and stroma in a lobulocentric configuration. Particularly in the center of such lesions, the stroma may compress and distort the acinar elements, producing a pattern that may mimic infiltrating carcinoma. Many examples of sclerosing adenosis are associated with calcifications that may be seen on mammograms.

Atypical hyperplasia Atypical hyperplasias are proliferative lesions of the breast that possess some, but not all, of the features of carcinoma *in situ*. Thus, an understanding of the histologic features of atypical hyperplasia requires familiarity with the histologic features of carcinoma *in situ*. Atypical hyperplasias are categorized as either ductal or lobular in type. *Atypical ductal hyperplasias* are lesions that have some of the architectural or cytologic features of ductal carcinoma *in situ*, such as nuclear monomorphism, regular cell placement, and round regular spaces, in at least part of the involved duct. Similarly, *atypical lobular hyperplasias* are characterized by changes similar to those of lobular carcinoma *in situ* but lack the complete criteria for that diagnosis. In addition to involving lobular units, the cells of atypical lobular hyperplasia may involve ducts.

Patients with atypical hyperplasia have a significantly increased risk of developing breast cancer. The risk of breast cancer for patients with atypical hyperplasia was 4.4 times that of the general population in a long-term study. Furthermore, among patients with atypical hyperplasia and a family history of breast cancer, the relative risk of subsequent breast cancer was 8.9, approaching that of patients with carcinoma *in situ*.

Other forms of benign disease

Benign neoplasms and proliferative lesions

Fibroadenomas These lesions are most commonly seen when palpable masses are biopsied. At the time of the procedure, fibroadenomas appear pseudoencapsulated and are sharply delineated from the surrounding breast tissues. They are usually spherical or singularly ovoid, but may be multilobulated. On cut section, the tumor bulges above the level of the surrounding breast tissue. The cut surface is most typically grey-white, and small, punctuate, yellow to pink soft areas and slitlike spaces are usually present. Fresh tumor may show a gelatinous, mucoid consistency.

Microscopically, fibroadenomas have both an epithelial and stromal component. The histologic pattern depends upon which of these components predominates. In general, the epithelial component consists of well-defined, glandlike and ductlike spaces lined by cuboidal or columnar cells with uniform nuclei. Varying degrees of epithelial hyperplasia are frequently observed. The stromal component consists of connective tissue that has a variable content of acid mucopolysaccharides and collagen.

These tumors occur more commonly in Blacks than in Caucasians. Typically, they appear during the active reproductive years, implicating some hormonal factor for their development. They often present a frightening gross clinical picture. Patients have a palpable mass which may occur with skin retraction or fixation to the pectoral muscle of the chest wall. This similarity of granular cell tumors to carcinoma is also appreciated on mammographic examination, on which they resemble scirrhous carcinoma. Grossly, the lesion shows a grey–white to tan firm tumor that may be gritty when cut with a knife; these features further support a diagnosis of carcinoma. Microscopically, several authors describe these lesions as being identical with granualar cell tumors in other sites, consisting of a poorly circumscribed proliferation of clusters of cells in which the most characteristic feature is prominent granularity of the cytoplasm.

Fibromatosis Fibromatosis of the breast is similar to fibromatosis elsewhere and is characterized by a locally invasive, non-encapsulated proliferation of well-differentiated fibroblasts. These tumors have the capacity to recur locally when inadequately removed, but they do not metastasize. Patients typically present with a palpable mass, which sometimes resembles fibroadenomas. On mammography, these lesions are indistinguishable from carcinomas and grossly when cut they are ill-defined, firm, grey–white lesions. The best treatment for these lesions is a wide local excision, since lesions do recur locally.

Benign tumors and related conditions

Lipomas consist of encapsulated nodules of mature adipose tissue. Although true lipomas occur in the breast, many lesions designated 'lipoma' probably represent foci of fatty breast tissue without a true capsule. Benign fatty tumors of the breast which contain entrapped lobular epithelial elements are called *adenolipomas*. The distinction between these lesions and breast tissues with prominent stromal adipose tissues is difficult to differentiate.

Leiomyomas of the breast are most often seen in the areolar region and rarely occur in the breast parenchyma. The histologic characteristics are the same as those of leiomyomas in the uterus and other tissues. *Neurofibromas* and *neurilemmomas (schwannomas)* are benign nerve sheath tumors. These areolar lesions are most frequently seen in the breast of those patients with neurofibromatosis. *Hamartomas* of the breast present as well-defined masses on physical examination and on mammography. Microscopically, they are composed of an admixture of ducts, lobules, fibrous stroma, and adipose tissue in varying proportions.

Juvenile fibroadenomas

Fibroadenomas in adolescents and younger women are generally similar to those in older patients, although a few which present a different clinical and pathologic picture are termed juvenile fibroadenomas.

Giant fibroadenomas

These tumors that are histologically typical fibroadenomas may often attain great size. Cystosarcoma phyllodes (preferably called a 'phyllodes tumor') is distinguished from a giant fibroadenoma by cellularity of the stromal component. Juvenile fibroadenomas may attain great sizes, and thus, may be variants of giant fibroadenomas.

Adenomas

Adenomas of the breast are well-circumscribed tumors composed of benign epithelial elements with sparse, inconspicuous stroma. The last feature is pathognomonic of adenomas and differentiates these lesions from the conspicuous stroma of the fibroadenomas.

Tubular adenomas, usually in young women, are well-defined and freely movable nodules clinically resembling fibroadenomas. On gross examination they show a well-circumscribed, tan-yellow, firm tumor, and on microscopic examination tubular adenomas are separated from the adjacent breast tissue by a pseudocapsule. The tubules comprise an inner epithelial layer and an outer myoepithelial layer resembling normal breast acini. The microscopic patterns are admixed with those of fibroadenomas, suggesting a relationship between the two tumor types.

Lactating adenomas appear as one or more freely movable masses during pregnancy or the postpartum period. They are grossly well circumscribed and lobulated and on cut section appear tan and softer than tubular adenomas. They appear as *de novo* lesions and are usually nodular foci of hyperplasia in the lactating breast.

Adenomas of the nipple Some adenomas of the nipple appear solid, grey–tan, and poorly demarcated tumors in the nipple and subareolar region. Often, no gross lesion is evident. Microscopically, the dominant feature is a proliferation of small glandlike structures. Reports of recurrence most likely represent cases in which the initial resection failed to remove the lesion completely.

Papillomas

Intraductal papillomas Several lesions in the breast are characterized by a papillary configuration seen grossly or microscopically. These include solitary intraductal papillomas, multiple (peripheral) papillomas, and papillomatosis. These are characterized clinically by an indistinct mass, with or without nipple discharge, and pathologically by multiple small but grossly evident papillary lesions.

Solitary intraductal papillomas are tumors of the major lactiferous ducts, most frequently observed in women ages 30–50 years. These lesions are generally small, less than 1 cm in diameter, usually measuring 3–4 mm. Rarely, they are as large as 4 or 5 cm. On gross examination, intraductal papillomas are tan–pink, friable tumors within a dilated duct or cyst.

Compared with solitary intraductal papillomas, *multiple intraductal papillomas* tend to occur in younger patients, are less often associated with nipple discharge, are more frequently peripheral, and are more often bilateral. These

lesions appear to be susceptible to the development of carcinoma, while no cases of carcinoma were found to be associated with solitary papillomas involving the large ducts. Peripheral papillomas, when compared to solitary central papillomas, are highly susceptible to malignant transformation.

Papillomatosis is defined as foci of hyperplasia that grows into a papillary configuration. Such lesions show the same significance as moderate or florid hyperplasia. The juvenile form of papillomatosis was first diagnosed in 1980. It occurs most commonly in adolescents and young women (with a mean age of 23 years) but has been described in women up to 48 years of age. Patients typically present with a painless mass that, on physical examination, is circumscribed, easily movable, and is most often considered to be a fibroadenoma. On gross examination, the mass ranges in size from 1 to 8 cm and multiple cysts of up to 1 cm in diameter are generally observed. Recent reports have suggested that juvenile papillomatosis is associated with an increased risk of breast cancer in the patient's female relatives and that the patient herself may be at increased risk for developing carcinoma.

Fat necrosis

The importance of fat necrosis is that it may closely simulate carcinoma, when viewed both clinically and on mammographic examination. The macroscopic appearance of fat necrosis depends on its age. In early lesions there is hemorrhage and indurated fat, while over time a rounded, firm tumor is formed. The cut surface of the lesion at this stage has a variegated, yellow–grey appearance, with focal hemorrhage. Cavitation may subsequently occur, owing to liquefactive necrosis. The lesion may eventually be converted to a dense, fibrous scar, or it may remain a cystic cavity with calcification of its walls.

Infarction

Fibroadenomas may undergo partial, subtotal, or total infarction. Pregnancy and lactation are the most common predisposing factors. It has been assumed that a relative vascular insufficiency due to increased metabolic activity in the breast underlies this phenomenon.

Reactions to foreign material

Foreign body-type granulomatous inflammation has been described following injection or implantation of a variety of substances, particularly silicone, within the breast for therapeutic, cosmetic or replacement purposes. Clinically, these lesions generally appear as multiple firm nodules that may be tender.

TREATMENT OF BENIGN BREAST DISEASES

Therapies for benign breast diseases, in general, have been limited to subjective symptoms. When pain is present, analgesics are given in various doses. The level of therapy is dependent on the extent of disruption of everyday activity that occurs. During the last two decades a series of medications have been used specifically for premenopausal women with breast pain. These antihormones reduce the cyclicity of the menstrual cycle and thus prevent hormonal fluctuations responsible for tissue enlargement, pain, secretion, and lumps in the breasts.

Benign breast nodules accompanied by pain (mastalgia) are present in 65–80% of all reproductive-aged women and 30% of this discomfort is in the perimenopausal period. While fibrocystic disease has been discussed and considered a misnomer for all mastalgias, this general term is referred to by most physicians on the basis of the symptoms of nodularity and discomfort. Cyclic breast pain occurs in 95% of all women with ovulatory cycles. The discomfort begins mildly after ovulation and continues to worsen for variable lengths of time until menses occurs with the average number of days cited as 5 ± 1.3 days.

The pain described may be localized or cover the total breast area. When mammography is done, it may show a range of findings from large multicystic clumps of tissue to no changes. The larger lesions may obscure tumors, particularly small carcinomas, which may lie behind them. For this reason, radiologists recommend postmenstrual studies which would eliminate the hormonal elements that occur. Large tender cysts are aspirated directly, which results in reducing discomfort and making mammograms more accurate. Several non-invasive therapies have been suggested before mammography to improve on this problem. When carcinoma has been fully ruled out as the cause of the symptoms present, a variety of maintenance treatments, described below, are usable.

Prophylactically, daily vitamins C and E, small doses of anti-prostaglandins and dietary avoidance of caffeine have been considered effective for many patients, particularly those with cyclic pain. None of these methods has been shown to have any scientific validity, but may individually provide relief.

Most treatments that have been recommended suppress active estrogen metabolism in the breast tissues. Many of the benign fibrocystic changes have pathognomonic findings of ductile/lobular hyperplasia, periductal fibrosis, increased ductal secretions with expanded cystic structures and adenosis of the cells with hypertrophy of the ducts. Experimentally, these have been shown to be produced by estrogen excess and/or with an increased prolactin stimulation. This has led to the use of drugs which are antiestrogenic and/or with a prolactin-lowering response.

Treatment with anti-estrogens such as Danocrine (danazol), tamoxifen citrate (Nolvadex) and gestrinone has resulted in improvement of benign fibrocystic changes diagnosed by tissue biopsy and mammograms. Pain has been relieved moderately by these anti-estrogenic substances. However, dosage levels are kept relatively low because of the marked side-effects described with the use of these products. Hormone treatment with progesterone shows variable success. Thyroid and cortisone hormone therapy has not been reliably effective.

Use of elemental iodine has produced a high level of improvement with reduced fibrosis.

Fibrocystic changes due to iodine deficiency were seen to increase with aging and were more responsive to replacement. These prescription therapies are presently in trial in both the United States and Canada. The side-effects appear to be minimal and a more accurate mammography may be obtainable, since the iodine therapy eliminates much of the nodularity and most of the fibrosis.

Birth control medications provide increased amounts of both estrogen and progesterone over the physiologic levels. When the cause of mastalgia is the menstrual cycle, this may be successful; however, when dose-related, little improvement may be seen.

Menopausal women who use oral estrogen–progestin replacement or estrogen alone therapy may notice increased breast size and occasional discomfort during the treatment. Those on oral estrogen–progesterone as a continuous regimen may develop larger breasts than those with estrogen therapy and several days of progestin monthly. Since the estrogen replacement therapy used contains less estrogen than premenopausal physiologic levels, the overall dosage does not seem to change breast cancer risk. Women with moderate to severe menopausal symptoms who have breast neoplasia or are at high risk for breast cancer are in a therapeutic dilemma. Progestational agents, clonidine, and tranquilizers have been suggested as a substitute for estrogen replacement therapy. Tamoxifen therapy is effective as an anti-estrogen and to decrease breast tenderness post-carcinoma. It often reduces osteoporosis present in the menopause as well, and would seem safer than estrogen replacement. When estrogen has been considered as absolutely contraindicated, recent studies have suggested that replacement is permissible if progestational therapy is used concurrently and estrogen receptor positive tumors are not involved. All replacement therapy requires the consent and understanding of the patient after personal evaluation of risks and benefits.

Bibliography

Cancer Committee of the College of American Pathologists. Is fibrocystic disease of the breast precancerous? *Arch Path Lab Med* 1986;110:171–3

Dupont WD, Page DL. Risk factors for breast cancer in women with proliferative breast disease. *N Engl J Med* 1985;312:146–51

Eskin BA. Malignant potential of benign breast lesions: indications for estrogen therapy. *J Am Med Assoc* 1991;266:1146

Ghent WR, Eskin BA, Low DA, *et al.* Iodine replacement in fibrocystic disease of the breast. *Can J Surg* 1993;36:453

London SJ, Connolly JL, Schmitt SJ, *et al.* A prospective study of benign breast disease and the risk of breast cancer. *J Am Med Assoc* 1992;267:941–2

Steinberg KK, Thacker SB, Smith JS, *et al.* A meta-analysis of the effect of estrogen replacement therapy and the risk of breast cancer. *J Am Med Assoc* 1991;265:1985–90

Fine needle aspiration cytology 11

P. Edmonds and L. Jardines

HISTORY OF FINE NEEDLE ASPIRATION (FNA) OF THE BREAST

Needle aspiration biopsy originated in Europe in the late 1800s. However, it was not used extensively for diagnostic purposes in breast disease in the United States and in Europe until the 1930s. In the post World War II era, concerns emerged regarding implantation of tumor following needle aspiration (especially with respect to sampling of lung tumors with large bore needles), and fine needle aspiration fell into decline in most centers. FNA was largely eclipsed as a diagnostic modality by frozen section during the 1950s and 60s. During this time, it was generally believed that 'a breast tumor should be excised to determine its nature with certainty, because the preoperative physical assessment had been subject to much uncertainty'. FNA did not re-emerge into wide acceptance until the late 1970s. In the past two decades, increasing acceptance of FNA has been driven by several factors: (1) cost containment pressures; (2) increasing movement of patient care out of hospital venues; (3) patient desire for a less disfiguring diagnostic procedure and, (4) conclusive evidence that spread of tumor by needle penetration prior to the definitive surgical treatment is not a clinical concern.

ROLE OF FNA IN PATIENT MANAGEMENT

The utilization of FNA as part of the initial evaluation of palpable breast masses has increased tremendously since it was rediscovered. The information gained from an aspiration may be of enormous value in guiding the need for further diagnostic and therapeutic maneuvers. Directed FNA of mammographically or ultrasonographically detected lesions is gaining acceptance in some centers, and is discussed in Chapter 5.

For FNA to play an important role in patient management, there must be a high level of confidence in the diagnoses rendered: both false-negative and false-positive reports must be minimized. Eliminating false-positive reports is the responsibility of the cytopathologist, and can be accomplished by strict adherence to diagnostic criteria for malignancy. It is the goal of cytopathology laboratories to have 0% false-positive diagnoses, so that clinicians can confidently proceed to definitive therapy based on the FNA diagnosis. In many large centers, the false-positive rate is under 1%.

False-negative diagnoses are more complex, and are much more common, ranging between 8% and 13.2% in two recent large series. One source of false-negative diagnoses is erroneous interpretation of cytologic material. Improved training of cytopathologists with board certification in this area has hopefully minimized such errors. Some particular entities, such as lobular carcinoma, are particularly difficult to recognize. A greater source of false-negative studies is the interpretation of samples as negative which are actually unsatisfactory. Criteria for a satisfactory FNA include a properly performed procedure, with adequate cellularity and preservation. If these criteria are not met, the sample must be termed unsatisfactory, not negative, and a repeat sample obtained, or an open biopsy performed if clinically indicated. Perhaps the most insidious form of false-negative study is one wherein a reasonably cellular sample is procured, with clearly benign cells, which nevertheless represents a 'geographic miss' of the lesion. A cytopathologist working in a vacuum, without adequate clinical information, cannot detect this sort of false-negative. These 'geographic miss' false-negative studies are likely to increase in the future, as rising patient and physician vigilance brings ever smaller breast masses to attention and work-up.

'Geographic miss' false negatives can be averted in two ways. One is by careful attention by the aspirator as to the textural quality of the mass as the needle is introduced. A crisp or gritty quality is typical of carcinomas, whereas many benign breast masses have a more rubbery quality. Failing to experience this gritty quality when aspirating a lesion which is otherwise highly suspicious for carcinoma could be a clue to a possible geographic miss. The other guard against false-negative studies is the so-called 'triple test', where FNA results are correlated with clinical impression and mammographic findings. If all three studies indicate that a lesion is benign, than the predictive value is comparable to that of open biopsy, and surgery can be confidently avoided. If all three studies indicate malignancy, then definitive therapy can be discussed with the patient with confidence. A surgical biopsy is indicated when there is a discrepancy in the findings of the triple test (for example, highly suspicious mammogram, malignant features on clinical exam, benign cytology). In women under 35 years of age who present with a palpable breast mass, a 'modified triple test' is recommended to determine the true nature of the lesion. In young women, where mammography is generally less helpful, a breast ultrasound directed to the site of the palpable finding is substituted for a mammogram. When directed breast ultrasound is combined with clinical breast exam and FNA, there is a high degree of sensitivity and specificity.

Approximately 80% of open surgical biopsies reveal benign disease. By employing the triple test strategy, the number of open biopsies performed can be reduced by 50% while maintaining a diagnostic sensitivity of 98.8%, which is comparable to frozen section. This represents substantial benefit in the form of greater patient satisfaction and convenience, and lower morbidity, as well as cost savings.

DIFFERENCES BETWEEN FNA AND CORE NEEDLE BIOPSY

Although a core needle biopsy and a fine needle aspiration biopsy have some obvious points in common (indeed, they may be indistinguishable from the patient's point of view), the practitioner should be aware of some important differences. Most FNAs are performed with a 21–25 gauge needle, rather than a cutting core needle (14 gauge). FNA and core needle biopsy also differ in the need for anesthesia prior to the procedure. Clinicians (usually surgeons) performing a core needle biopsy almost invariably use local anesthetic on the skin and soft tissue overlying the target lesion. While some practitioners also use local anesthesia prior to an FNA, others feel that the puncture to administer the anesthesia is as painful as the procedure itself, and, therefore, of limited value. The most salient difference, from the pathologist's point of view, is the nature of the sample obtained. The core needle biopsy procures a core of tissue which requires overnight processing, paraffin embedding and sectioning to produce a slide for viewing which provides histology.

FNA procures a suspension of disaggregated cells rather than a core of tissue. This suspension can be directly smeared on slides, which is the fastest method. Alternatively, the cell suspension can be expelled into a liquid fixative medium, for subsequent preparation by a variety of techniques, all of which take less than one hour. Consequently, same-day diagnosis is frequently possible. Core needle biopsies have the advantage of allowing better evaluation of architecture and of the relationship of the epithelial cells to the surrounding stroma. While cytologic criteria exist to distinguish between invasive and *in-situ* carcinoma, most pathologists agree that this distinction is more reliably made on tissue biopsy than by cytology. Both FNA and core needle biopsy have a higher false-negative rate based in sampling artifact (geographic miss), than that of open surgical biopsy. It has been argued that FNA may actually have a lower geographic miss rate than core needle biopsy, because the 'fanning' technique of changing needle angle allows sampling of a wider area than a core. Finally, core biopsies and FNAs differ in the amount of material obtained for ancillary studies. Although procedures exist to perform estrogen and progesterone receptor (ER/PR) assays and ploidy studies on FNA samples, core biopsies usually provide more material for ancillary studies.

TECHNIQUE OF FNA

Localization of the target

The first step in FNA of breast masses is defining the target lesion, and its relationship to surrounding structures. The depth of the lesion within the breast (the distance from the skin surface) will determine the length of the needle needed to reach the target. The relationship of the target lesion to the chest wall may be of importance in the ability successfully to immobilize the lesion. Target lesions close to or immediately beneath the nipple may present particular problems in performing the FNA comfortably since the skin of the nipple and areola is extremely sensitive. It is recommended that subareolar masses be approached obliquely rather than through the nipple or areola.

Equipment

Needle

The length of the needle required is dictated by the depth of the target. The needle employed should be no longer than necessary, as a longer more flexible needle risks a degree of 'wobble'.

The gauge of the needle employed is in part a matter of personal preference, but most aspirators use between a 21 and a 25 gauge. Smaller gauge needles may not retrieve an adequate sample, and also risk distortion of the sample by shear effect. Larger gauge needles are unnecessarily uncomfortable, and may extract actual tissue core biopsies which, while well suited for embedding and sectioning, produce smears which are too thick to be properly evaluated.

Syringe

A 10 ml syringe is generally adequate to provide the needed suction to draw the sample into the needle. When aspirating a solid mass, at the completion of the procedure the sample should be contained in the needle and the hub of the needle. It is a misconception that the syringe will be filled, even partially, by the sample. On occasion, a cystic lesion may provide several milliliters of fluid filling, or partially filling the syringe. Even so, syringes larger than 10 ml are seldom needed to adequately evacuate a cyst.

Syringe holder

A variety of pistol grip type syringe holders are available which can facilitate directing the needle and maintaining proper suction at the same time. These are especially helpful for aspirators with small or weak hands.

Performing the aspiration

Having localized and immobilized the mass, and cleansed the overlying skin with alcohol, the barrel of the syringe is pulled back to the 0.5–1 ml mark and the needle is inserted through the skin into the mass. Suction is applied and excursions are made through the mass with the needle. Some authors have advocated a chipping or ice pick-like motion. Aspirators differ as to whether the angle of the needle should be altered during the excursions, moving the needle through the tissue in a 'fanning', arc-like pattern. While changing the angle of the needle widens the field that is sampled, it also increases the risk of bleeding, which may dilute and obscure the sample. Even if the needle angle is altered during aspirations, all authors agree that at minimum two to four passes should be made to reduce the risk of missing the target. After 10 or 15 excursions of the needle, suction is released and the needle is withdrawn. It is a very important factor (and one often overlooked) that suction must be released while the needle is still in the target. Otherwise, the sample will be drawn out of the needle and into the syringe, where it is more difficult to expel onto the slide, and where air-drying immediately begins to take place. With the release of the suction, the barrel of the syringe will return to the preset location and will provide the necessary air to expel the material onto the slide or into the fixative.

Specimen handling

At the conclusion of the aspiration, the sample should be contained in the needle itself, and the needle hub. Two main options are available to transfer the sample to glass slides for interpretation; fluid fixation and/or direct smears. During the process of fluid fixation, the sample is expelled into liquid fixative or transport medium for subsequent processing in the laboratory. This processing may include direct smears, but more likely is a concentration technique such as cytospin, filter, or Thin prep® preparation, depending on the resources and preferences of the laboratory. Fluid fixation is probably the simplest and most reliable method for obtaining consistent results. It is recommended for aspirators who have limited experience preparing direct smears, and who work without an assistant. Several studies have shown that preparations from fluid fixatives are equally as diagnostic as direct smears.

To prepare a direct smear, a droplet of sample is placed on a glass slide and smeared, analogous to preparing a smear of peripheral blood. The smear must be immediately fixed if it is to be stained with Papanicolaou stain (the standard in most cytology laboratories). Air drying of as little as 15 s can compromise quality. Many pathologists prefer direct smears for their better demonstration of cellular architecture, of background material, and for their speed of preparation. A poorly prepared smear, one which is overly thick, overly thin, dried, or obscured by blood or inflammation, is often inferior to a fluid preparation. Many laboratories can send personnel to the bedside in hospital, or to clinics, to assist with the preparation of smears. However, as more care is delivered outside of the hospital setting, the availability of such assistance may be limited in the future.

Specimen adequacy

The issue of specimen adequacy in breast cytology is of critical importance, because a significant number of 'false-negative' samples are truly inadequate samples. Unfortunately, a definition of adequacy is somewhat elusive for breast aspirates. Moriarty defines an adequate specimen as 'one which depicts the abnormality which is present'. Although it is difficult to argue with this definition, it necessarily follows that many different cytologic findings may all represent adequate samples, dependent on the different underlying lesions from which they were derived. For example, blood, with few epithelial elements, may represent an adequate sample of a hematoma, but not of a solid mass mammographically suspicious of carcinoma. The differing nature of target lesions in part frustrates our attempts to assign a single quantitative standard of adequacy to all specimens. However, some guidelines are useful.

The minimum number of passes required to constitute an adequate sample is two to four; most authors agree that a single pass is seldom adequate. One of the authors (L.J.) routinely makes 15–20 passes through the target lesion provided the patient is not too uncomfortable. Several passes are encouraged both for small and for large target lesions; for small lesions so as to ensure that a geographic miss does not occur, and for large lesions so as to sample different areas in a potentially heterogeneous target. The number of ductal epithelial cells necessary for adequacy is four to six cell groups, each consisting of six to ten cells. Less cellular samples are considered inadequate by virtue of insufficient cellularity. An aspirate is considered adequate only if specimen handling is appropriate to allow interpretation; air-drying, obscuring blood or inflammation must not interfere with the diagnosis. Otherwise, even a sufficiently cellular sample can be rendered inadequate. Finally, a sample cannot be considered adequate if the cytologic diagnosis is at odds with that expected based on clinical examination and imaging studies, even if the above criteria are met. An inadequate sample requires either a repeat aspiration, or an open biopsy. An inadequate sample must never be interpreted as equivalent of negative.

Communication with the laboratory

Communication implies a two-way dialogue; clinicians need information from the laboratory in the form of diagnoses, provided in a timely fashion, and laboratories need information from the clinicians in the form of clinical history, physical examination and mammographic findings, to aid in the interpretation of the cytologic sample. In the European system, where the person performing the aspiration also interprets it, such communication is unnecessary; where these responsibilities are divided, it is essential.

As with all laboratory samples, accurate specimen identification is the first step. Patient name and age are minimal demographics. As discussed earlier, information regarding the mass itself are critical to recognition of discrepancies between cytologic features and clinical expectations. Size of the mass, location, duration, variation in size with menses, pain, mobility, fixation to skin or chest wall, and associated nipple discharge are all useful pieces of information.

Results from FNA procedures can often be available on the day of the procedure. The most rapid results are obtained from material processed by direct smear, at the site where the FNA was performed, which can provide a diagnosis essentially on a 'while you wait' basis. Additional time is required if material is fixed in fluid fixative for subsequent spin or filter preparations. If the specimen is transported to a central laboratory, logistics of pick-up and delivery may factor considerably into the time required to deliver the results. Return of the report to the source can be either by courier, or, increasingly by fax. Most laboratories have a policy of notification by phone for all malignant diagnoses rendered.

INTERPRETING THE FNA DIAGNOSES

Increasingly, as our diagnostic criteria improve, specific diagnoses are rendered, similar to those made by open biopsy. Some of the specific pathologic entities which can be diagnosed by FNA are discussed below. Even if a specific diagnosis is not made, cytologic findings should be categorized into five basic groups:

Basic cytologic categories

1. Unsatisfactory: this is the equivalent in the work-up strategy of 'no sample' and this means that too few ductal epithelial cells have been obtained to provide a diagnosis.

2. Benign: the cells obtained meet none of the cytologic criteria of malignancy. These can be derived from normal parenchyma or benign lesions such as fibrocystic changes or fibroadenoma.

3. Atypical: cells which, while probably benign, show some abnormal features, including nuclear enlargement, nucleoli, etc. A small number of these cases may prove to be carcinoma, but most probably are derived from epithelial hyperplasia in fibrocystic changes.

4. Suspicious: cells with many, but not all, features of malignancy. A high proportion of these cases will prove, on biopsy, to be

carcinoma. However, in cases called suspicious, the level of certainty is insufficient to proceed to definitive treatment without an open biopsy. As we strive to reduce false-positive diagnoses to zero, suspicious calls necessarily rise and include some low histologic grade carcinomas.

5. Malignant: cells meet all criteria of malignancy. Definitive therapy may be planned based on this diagnosis.

Specific benign diagnoses

Fibroadenomas are common lesions, with a distinctive cytomorphologic pattern (Figure 11.1) Groups of ductal epithelial cells appear as branching, cohesive, 'stag-horn' groups. The fibrous stroma is represented as single bipolar nuclei, without apparent cytoplasm. This cytologic picture, coupled with the distinctive clinical and mammographic appearance is usually diagnostic, although some individual cases may present diagnostic problems.

The cellular elements of fibrocystic changes (FCC) are highly heterogeneous on biopsy, and similarly so on aspiration. One of the most characteristic features of FCC is apocrine metaplasia. The apocrine metaplastic cells, with their abundant granular eosinophilic cytoplasm and their large but uniform nucleoli, are easily recognized, especially when coupled with foamy histiocytes, which are usually seen in cyst contents. More difficult diagnostically are the epithelial elements, especially when hyperplasia is prominent. Attempts to correlate cytologic findings with histologic findings in ductal hyperplasia with and without atypia have not been productive so far.

Malignant diagnoses

The majority of malignant diagnoses made are of ductal carcinoma (Figure 11.2). Several criteria go into making this cytologic diagnosis and no single parameter predicts malignancy reliably. The cytologic findings that are evaluated and which correspond with malignancy

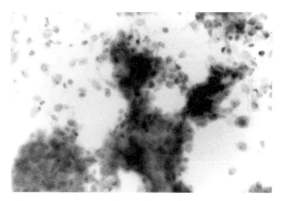

Figure 11.1 Fibroadenoma with 'staghorn' clusters of uniform epithelial cells and singly arrayed stromal cells in the background (Papanicolaou stain, original magnification ×25)

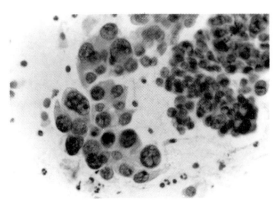

Figure 11.2 Ductal carcinoma with highly pleomorphic cells which exhibit variability in nuclear size and prominent nucleoli (hematoxylin and eosin stain, original magnification ×25)

are: increased cellularity, dyshesion, the increased size and variability of the size of the nucleus, prominence of the nucleoli, a coarse chromatin pattern, and an irregular nuclear membrane. When most or all of these criteria are met, a malignant diagnosis can be made with confidence.

Lobular carcinoma shares some of the diagnostic features of ductal carcinoma; indeed, studies suggest that they cannot always be reliably distinguished. Marked dyshesion is present, and chromatin pattern is abnormal, but cells of lobular carcinoma are typically smaller and less variable in size, therefore less eye-catching, leading to a diagnostic pitfall.

Tubular, mucinous, and papillary carcinoma are histologic subtypes of ductal carcinoma. Distinctive cytomorphometric features (pointed ductal structures, mucinous background material, papillary architecture) may allow for their specific identification. All have a relatively low degree of pleomorphism, which can make distinction from benign entities more difficult.

Limitations of FNA diagnosis

Although specific diagnostic accuracy is improving with FNA, certain important limits compared to histologic diagnosis must be recognized. Because the diagnosis of invasion is predicated on breach of the basement membrane, cytology cannot reliably make this distinction. Ductal carcinoma *in situ* with marked cytologic atypia (comedo carcinoma) can have a degree of pleomorphism equal to invasive carcinomas. It can be difficult to make a definitive diagnosis of carcinoma of a low histologic grade. Because a malignant diagnosis is made based on recognition of abnormal nuclear features, low histologic grade carcinomas which have minimal nuclear abnormality may be difficult to diagnose. Occasionally, only some of the more subtle features of malignancy may be present, such as increased cellularity and dyshesion. In these cases, a report of suspicious for carcinoma with open biopsy recommended is prudent.

Features in FCC which are associated with a higher risk of carcinoma include ductal hyperplasia, especially if florid or atypical. These entities are difficult to recognize cytologically, as they share features with both non-proliferative breast disease and with those types of ductal carcinoma *in situ* where cytologic atypia is minimal (cribriform and micropapillary). It is hardly surprising that this distinction is difficult cytologically, as these lesions are challenging to distinguish on histologic grounds as well.

COMPLICATIONS OF FNA

Morbidity from FNA is extremely low and mortality unknown. Infectious risk can be eliminated by proper cleansing of the skin prior to aspiration. Untoward bleeding is rarely encountered, and can be controlled by appropriate application of pressure. Rare reports exist of pneumothorax occurring when the chest wall is penetrated when performing FNA in the breast. Early concerns regarding dissemination of disease by puncture prior to excision have been allayed. The final concern, raised more recently in the pathology literature, is of obscuring of the lesion, when ultimately excised, by artifacts imposed by puncture. In several cases, displaced fragments of epithelium have been attributed to needle puncture; however, this is seen more often with core needle biopsies than with FNA. These fragments have the potential to be misinterpreted as spread of tumor. As pathologists are alerted to this phenomenon, their ability to recognize it should improve.

CONCLUSION

Fine needle aspiration biopsy is a simple, safe, rapid, diagnostic procedure which has considerable value in the outpatient management of palpable breast masses. Increased operator experience and close communication with the laboratory providing interpretation can maximize the benefits for patients. It is important to interpret the results of the cytologic diagnosis in conjunction with the remainder of the clinical evaluation. A negative cytology report should not dissuade one from proceeding with open surgical biopsy if clinical breast exam and/or imaging studies are suspicious.

Bibliography

Hermansen C, Poulsen HS, Jensen J, *et al.* Diagnostic reliability of combined physical examination, mammography, and fine-needle puncture ('Triple-Test') in breast tumors: a prospective study. *Cancer* 1987;60:1866–71

Howat AJ, Stringfellow HF, Briggs WA, *et al.* Fine needle aspiration cytology of the breast: a review of 1868 cases using the cytospin method. *Acta Cytol* 1994;38:939–45

Kline TS. Survey of aspiration biopsy cytology of the breast. *Diagn Cytopathol* 1991;7:98–105

Layfield LJ. Can fine-needle aspiration replace open biopsy in the diagnosis of palpable breast lesions? *Am J Clin Pathol* 1992;98:145–7

Masood S. Cytopathology of the breast; ASCP theory and practice of cytopathology. Chicago: ASCP Press, 1996:1–429

Moriarty A. Fine-needle biopsy of the breast: when is enough, enough? *Diagn Cytopathol* 1995;13:373–4

Sneige N, Fornage BN, Saleh G. Ultrasound-guided fine-needle aspiration of non-palpable breast lesions: cytologic and histologic findings. *Am J Clin Pathol* 1994;102:98–101

Sneige N, Staerkel GA, Caraway NP, *et al.* A plea for uniform terminology and reporting of breast fine needle aspirates: the M.D. Anderson Cancer Center Proposal. *Acta Cytol* 1994;38:971–2

Sneige N. Fine-needle aspiration of the breast: a review of 1995 cases with emphasis on diagnostic pitfalls. *Diagn Cytopathol* 1993;9:106–12

Vetto J, Pommier R, Schmidt WA, *et al.* Use of the 'triple test' for palpable breast lesions yields high diagnostic accuracy and cost savings. *Am J Surg* 1995;169:519–22

Vetto JT, Pommier RF, Schmidt WA, *et al.* Diagnosis of palpable breast lesions in younger women by the modified triple test is accurate and cost-effective. *Arch Surg* 1996;131:967–74

Willis, SL, Ramzy I. Analysis of false results in a series of 835 fine needle aspirates of breast lesions. *Acta Cytol* 1995;39:858–64

Youngson BJ, Cranor M, Rosen PP. Epithelial displacement in surgical breast specimens following needling procedures. *Am J Surg Pathol* 1994;18:896–903

Pathology of common premalignant and malignant lesions of the breast

12

I. Daskal

INTRODUCTION

The intention of this chapter is to provide the primary care physician with a broad overview of the pathology of the premalignant lesions and common malignancies of the breast and some of the relationships between the histology and the biology of the lesions. The emphasis is on those lesions which the family practitioner is most likely to encounter in his daily practice. The pathology of lesions of low prevalence such as less than 1% is not addressed. For example, although angiosarcoma of the breast is biologically a very aggressive lesion with poor outcome, it is of low prevalence (<0.2%) and, hence, was excluded from this review.

The discussion of prognostic indicators and risk factors for breast cancer are discussed in great detail in Chapter 19. The management of breast cancers is discussed in Chapters 14–16.

This chapter will review, in addition to the salient morphological features of the more frequent malignant breast lesions, some epidemiological and prognostic data where appropriate. For the reader who wants to pursue the subject to greater depth, a suggested reading list, consisting of important recent texts on the subject, is included at the end of the chapter.

PREMALIGNANT LESIONS OF THE BREAST

Numerous epidemiological studies have attempted to show the existence of precursor lesions as the transition state between normal breast tissue and carcinoma. For example, a continuum consisting of hyperplasia, to atypical hyperplasia to frank carcinoma was targeted to fit into such a model. Hence, atypical hyperplasia of the breast clearly connotes those histological features which could yield significant risks for the patient to progress towards the development of carcinoma. The recognition of this transition between atypical hyperplasia and carcinoma has important prognostic implications. Unfortunately, the diagnosis of atypical hyperplasia, as will be discussed below, poses a significant problem due to observer subjectivity and less than rigid criteria for its recognition.

The term hyperplasia suggests an increase of the number of cells in relationship to the basement membrane on which the cells rest. Therefore, an increase of three or more cells counted from the basement membrane towards the lumen is defined as hyperplasia. The basic micro-anatomy of the breast consists of two major components, the ducts and the lobules, both of which yield different hyperplastic lesions which will be described below.

Intraductal hyperplasia

Epidemiology and clinical presentation

These lesions may present clinically as a mass or an area of induration. These are commonly seen over a broad age range, starting from the second to the seventh decade of life. Mammographically, these may be interpreted as suspicious for malignancy despite the absence of micro-calcifications. Women with moderate to severe intraductal hyperplasia have approximately a two-fold increase in risk for the development of breast cancer.

Commonly, intraductal hyperplasia would not present grossly as an identifiable lesion. However, when associated with microcalcifications, it may present as a mammographic abnormality. When associated with significant fibrosis, the lesion may become palpable.

Histological presentation

Microscopically, one or more ducts may be involved. The proliferating epithelial cells may increase focally in number above the basement membrane (>3) or totally occlude the duct lumen leading to duct distention. Several patterns can be recognized, such as forming secondary lumens, tortuous ribbons of cells or micro-papillary patterns. Several microscopic features point towards a benign nature of the lesion:

1. Prominent layer of myoepithelial cells.

2. Presence of a heterogeneous population of cells; namely, epithelial, myoepithelial, and apocrine.

3. Mitotic figures and nucleoli may be present; however, cytologically the nuclei are not bizarre and atypical mitoses are not present.

4. Presence of foamy histiocytes in lumina without true lumen necrosis.

5. The micro-architecture of secondary lumens are variable in size and are oval, slit-like, or serrated configurations.

Prognosis

The degree of simple ductal hyperplasia is usually related to the cellularity of the lesions, reflecting a quantitative progression. Lesions, up to three or four cells thick, resting on the basement membrane, are classified as duct ectasia or mild hyperplasia. These do not confer increased risk for the development of invasive carcinoma. Even when micropapillary forms are present, these are not associated with increased risk. When the cellularity increases to more layers, reaching the opposing luminal border, these may be considered as moderate or florid hyperplasias, depending on the extent and severity of the changes. These patients were shown to have approximately two-fold risk over that of the general population for developing invasive breast carcinoma. As the histology continues to deviate from the normal, with forms resembling that of carcinoma, such as abnormal mitoses, increased monotonicity of the cells, resulting in atypical intraductal hyperplasia (AIH, see below), the risk may be as high as four-to five-fold of the normal population. Moderate to florid hyperplasias may be encountered in approximately 20% of all breast biopsies.

Atypical intraductal hyperplasia

The diagnosis of atypical intraductal hyperplasia in the breast in relation to proliferative lesions should be interpreted as a premalignant state, especially in a patient with a family history of breast cancer. Being defined as the transitional lesion towards frank carcinoma magnifies the need for adequate objective morphologic criteria to recognize this lesion, and hence, identify patients with increased risks of developing invasive carcinoma.

The risk of carcinoma was increased in either breast when atypical hyperplasia was diagnosed in the contralateral breast. Conversely, atypical hyperplasia is more commonly found when carcinomas present in the contralateral breast.

An important contribution towards a criterion based diagnosis of atypical hyperplasia was made by DuPont and Page. They concluded that 'atypical hyperplasia shares some but not all of the features of carcinoma in situ (CIS).' They have shown that women with atypical hyperplasia (AIH) had a 5.3-fold increased risk of developing invasive cancer over the general population. Tavassoli and Norris have shown, in a study of 200 women with the diagnosis of AIH, approximately 10% of the patients progressed and developed invasive carcinoma. In women with familial risk factors in addition to AIH, the risks are doubled.

Histopathology

A great deal of subjectivity still persists in the diagnosis of atypical hyperplasia despite numerous attempts to develop clear, rigid diagnostic criteria. Black and Chabon defined atypical hyperplasia as a 'linear progression process which culminates in carcinoma'. Thus, if the linear process consists of five grades, with grade 1 representing simple hyperplasia and carcinoma as grade 5, then atypical hyperplasia may manifest itself as multi-layering of cells, loss of nuclear polarity, increased nuclear cytoplasmic ratio and the presence of prominent nucleoli.

DuPont and Page, on the other hand, believed that the hyperplasia should differ from frank carcinoma, mostly on a quantitative basis; namely, 'the criteria for atypical hyperplasia should be derived from their corresponding carcinomas *in situ*.' Two major criteria are cited by these authors for the diagnosis of ductal carcinoma *in situ* (DCIS).

First, a monomorphic population of cells must fill a basement membrane enclosed space. Two such spaces are the minimal diagnostic criteria and, secondly, rigid arches and hyperchromatic nuclei are diagnostic prerequisites for DCIS. Therefore, AIH will be diagnosed when these elements of DCIS are present, but not completely.

Tavassoli and Norris expanded on the diagnostic criteria proposed by DuPont and Page. They recommend that a lesion to be diagnosed as intraductal carcinoma should measure in aggregate at least 2 mm in size. Smaller foci, although having histological features of carcinoma diagnostic of intraductal carcinoma, must be considered as intraductal atypical hyperplasia (Figure 12.1).

The most important feature to separate intraductal hyperplasia from atypical hyperplasia rests in the cytological characteristics of the cells in the absence of architectural organization of carcinoma. Therefore, when the classical monotonous features of an intraductal carcinoma are present, but the architecture is that of an intraductal hyperplasia, the lesion is considered by Tavassoli as atypical intraductal hyperplasia. The principle being that both the qualitative (cytology and architecture) and quantitative (lesion greater than 2 mm) criteria must be met for a diagnosis of carcinoma, otherwise these lesions should be considered as atypical intraductal hyperplasia. According to the authors 'it is important that the diagnosis of atypical intraductal hyperplasia should not be rendered when the pathologist is unable to decide whether the lesion represents an intraductal hyperplasia or carcinoma but only when the above diagnostic criteria are applied'.

Prognosis

As stated above, numerous studies have confirmed the increased risk for the development of invasive carcinoma in patients with AIH. The general agreement at present is that AIH carries a moderate risk of 4–5 times over that of the general population. In an extensive study of approximately 10 000 breast biopsies, DuPont and Page in 1989 determined that there is approximately 5% risk for invasive cancer in patients with AIH. It is hoped that molecular markers such as oncogene activation/expression or accurate measurements of the DNA content of the AIH will allow the development of objective criteria for the diagnosis of lesions with malignant potential.

PATHOLOGY OF MALIGNANT LESIONS

Non-infiltrating carcinomas

Non-infiltrating or *in situ* lesions are defined as malignant lesions confined to their original histological structure. In the breast, this represents any portion of the duct and/or lobular system. The confinement implies that the malignant cells have not violated the basement membrane complex and did not spill over into the

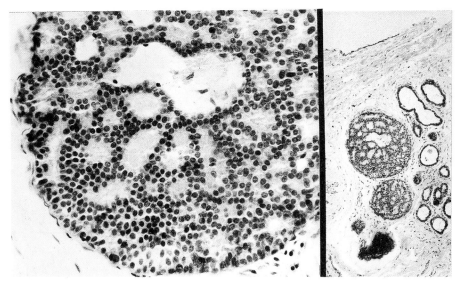

Figure 12.1 The lesion found in a lumpectomy of a 47-year-old woman is seen in the inset (×78). It consists of two ducts. At high magnification (main figure, ×780), it can be seen that it contains many of the features of ductal carcinoma *in situ*. Some arches appear less rigid at the periphery although nuclei are monotonous. Most of the secondary lumens are rounded. Using the criteria proposed by Page *et al.* this lesion would be diagnosed as DCIS since two ducts are involved. However, since in aggregate it measures less than 2 mm, it would qualify only for an ADH by the criteria recommended by Tavassoli

surrounding stroma. Significant controversy exists as to whether the *in situ* designation implies an intermediate stage leading to the evolution of a fully invasive lesion. At present, there is limited clinical and experimental data to support such a 'progressive theory' for the *in situ* lesions. Such considerations of the invasive potential of these lesions may have important treatment implications.

Intraductal carcinoma

Epidemiology and clinical presentation Intraductal carcinomas consist of a group of heterogeneous lesions as documented by molecular and clinical data. The histological patterns are variable and consist of a comedo, cribriform, clinging (micropapillary), papillary, solid and any combination of the above. The frequency of intraductal carcinoma ranges from 3 to 8% of the total tumors and approximately 50 to 70% of the total non-invasive lesions. Most of

these lesions are not palpable, the exception being the comedo carcinomas which yield a firmness which represents the expansion of the ducts with necrotic debris and cancer cells. These lesions are commonly identified by mammography as suspicious calcifications primarily in comedo carcinomas. However, 10–20% false-positive mammographic rate has been reported.

The mean age of diagnosis is in the fifth decade of life. A 25% incidence of occult carcinoma was reported. In about 30–40% of patients, mixed histological variants are present.

Comedo carcinoma

Gross and histological presentation The site of origin of this lesion is thought to be the terminal duct. The name comedo originates from the characteristic feature of the gross presentation of this lesion. When the cut surface is compressed, necrotic intraductal debris is expressed, which is reminiscent of comedos.

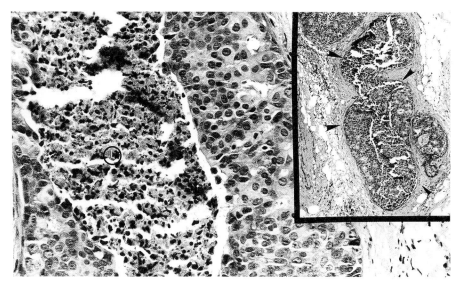

Figure 12.2 Intraductal carcinoma comedo type grade 2 (×780). Note some pleomorphism of the nuclei with some occasional nucleoli. Luminal (L) necrosis is present. Note the characteristic peri-ductal fibrosis (inset, ×78) and elastosis (pointers)

Histologically, these lesions consist of highly pleomorphic cells surrounding a lumen filled with necrotic debris (Figure 12.2). Some lesions consist of a solid or a cribriform pattern. This feature should be noted even when a single duct has a classical feature in the presence of other histological patterns. Myoepithelial cells are present, and the malignant cells may exhibit a brisk mitotic rate. A desmoplastic reaction accompanied by reactive lymphocytosis can be seen frequently. The distinction between necrosis and luminal secretion deposits must be made for the correct diagnosis of comedo carcinoma. The luminal duct contents in comedo carcinoma contain primarily ghosts of malignant cells and dystrophic calcifications. In contrast, luminal secretions contain mostly foamy macrophages and inflammatory cells. Of all the known invasive carcinomas, the comedo variant has the highest propensity for axillary node and systemic metastasis.

Cribriform variant This variant consists of groups of tumor cells which are monomorphic, haphazardly distributed throughout the duct and forming secondary lumens separated by rigid 'Roman bridges' (Figure 12.3). Usually, these cellular arches are at least two cells thick. The resulting fenestrations have round contours and are distributed throughout the duct. This is in contrast to atypical hyperplasias, which also contain monomorphic cells, but these form secondary lumina which are slit-like or highly scalloped, yielding the ribboning or streaming effect. Myoepithelial cells are frequently absent in this variant.

Clinging carcinoma (micropapillary) variant This variant was coined by Azopardi as 'clinging carcinoma'. It consists of a discontinuous layer of few cells which protrude into the luminal portion of the duct in an attempt to form secondary but incomplete fenestrations. These excrescences may consist of a few cells with 'hobnailed appearance' or form long slender processes. Some of these fronds may join to form thin 'Roman bridges' and secondary lumens, closely mimicking a cribriform pattern. Cytologically, the cells are monomorphic with low mitotic grade. Myoepithelial cells may be absent or discontinuous and replaced by tumor cells.

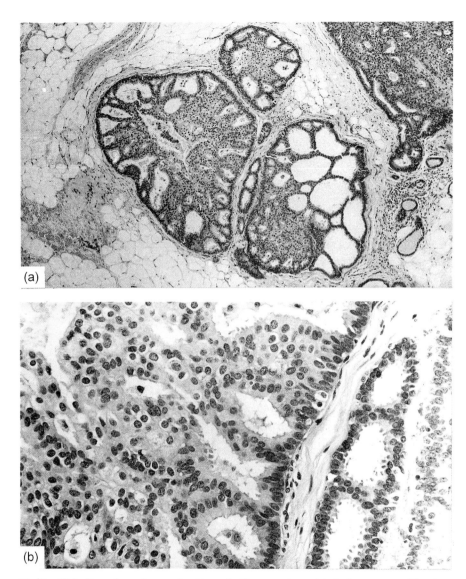

Figure 12.3 Ductal carcinoma *in situ*, cribriform variant. (a) At lower magnification (×400) the characteristic 'Roman bridges' are present. (b) At high magnification (×780) the haphazard arrangement of cells is seen. Note the low nuclear grade in this lesion

Papillary carcinoma

Epidemiology and clinical presentation The most common presentation of centrally located papillary carcinoma is that of a nipple discharge which may be bloody or blood-tinged. The majority of the lesions are palpable and may ulcerate. In about a third of patients, nipple retraction occurs. Multifocal peripheral lesions involving distal ducts and terminal lobular units are not usually palpable. This lesion can occur in males as well (Figure 12.4).

Gross and histopathological presentation Grossly, these tumors may appear to reside in dilated space, are friable and hemorrhagic. Papillary

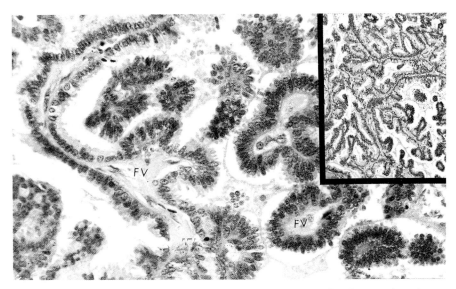

Figure 12.4 Papillary carcinoma (×780). The characteristics of an intracystic or intraductal papillary carcinoma are seen in the inset (×78). The long fronds contain a central supportive fibrovascular core (FV)

fronds may be identified. Microscopically, these consist of epithelial cells organized around a fibrovascular core within a distended duct (Figure 12.4). Some calcification may be present. Cytologically, the cells appear monotonous with occasional atypia. Mitotic rate may be brisk. An important diagnostic feature is the absence of a myoepithelial layer in the affected duct.

Solid intraductal carcinoma This pattern consists of tumor cells totally filling the duct lumen with or without calcifications. Necrosis is not a common feature, although focally it may be present. Cytologically, the nuclei are monomorphic, although cytoplasmic tinctorial quality varies. Myoepithelial cell layers are absent and, hence, the diagnostic feature for this entity. Other morphological variants, such as clear cell, signet cells, apocrine, spindle cells, and endocrine, are less common entities and their description is beyond the scope of this chapter.

Prognosis and grading of DCIS As early as the end of the 19th century, Hansenman, who

coined the term 'anaplasia', realized that the outcome of a malignancy is highly related to its morphological characteristics. During the last 70 years, it became clear that histological grading of tumors, especially in the breast, can predict outcome independent of disease stage. Although a grading system is widely accepted in invasive breast carcinomas, a unified methodology for grading DCIS is not yet available.

Several prognostic classification systems were proposed based on nuclear grade, differentiation, mitotic index, and a comedo type of necrosis. It is not totally clear what is the contribution of each of these components towards the final grade. Recently, Silverstein *et al.* proposed a novel classification system based on nuclear grade and the absence or presence of necrosis. The lesions were divided into two major categories: high grade and non-high grade.

High grade lesions (grade 3) were defined as those with high nuclear grades with or without a comedo pattern or necrosis. They observed that the nuclear grade alone was a strong predictor for the aggressiveness of this lesion.

Grade 2 lesions were those with necrosis but non-high grade nuclei. Lesions without necrosis

Table 12.1 Van Nuys prognostic index scoring system (from Silverstein MJ, *et al. The Breast Journal* 1996;2: 38–40)

Score	1	2	3
Size (mm)	<15	16–40	>41
Margins	>10	1–9	<1
Path. grade	1	2	3

were classified as grade 1. Using this grading system for DCIS (Van Nuys System), Silverstein was able to show a strong correlation between the grading system and probability for local recurrence. The higher the grade the higher the probability for recurrence.

Furthermore, by assigning a numerical value to the lesion size, histological grade and the distance of the lesion from the resected margins, Silverstein recommended an Index Score [Van Nuys Prognostic Index (VNPI)] system (Table 12.1) which was shown to be predictive of disease-free survival in his patients. The VNPI scoring system ranges from a low of 3 to a high of 9.

Patients with a VNPI score of 3–4 treated with breast conservation showed a disease-free survival of approximately 100% at 5 years. These patients most likely would not benefit from additional irradiation treatments. However, patients with intermediate scores (5, 6 or 7) following breast conservation had a DFS of 85% following irradiation, while patients with VNPI of 8 or 9 had an unacceptable recurrence rate with a DFS of only 20% with clear recommendation by the Van Nuys study for mastectomy.

Other histological grading systems using similar numerical values for mitotic rate, nuclear grade, margin involvement and glandular differentiation have been proposed in lieu of the Van Nuys classification but have not been widely accepted yet.

Mention must be made of the concept of 'microinvasion'. This refers to a microscopic violation of the basement membrane complex by malignant cells into the stroma. Although no rigid guidelines exist concerning the definition of 'microinvasion', it is generally accepted that such a focus is not to exceed 1 mm and should comprise less than 10% of the area studied. Some data suggests that up to 20% of patients with DCIS with 'microinvasion' will have lymph node involvement.

Lobular carcinoma in situ (LCIS)

Epidemiology and clinical presentation The incidence of LCIS is estimated at approximately 4–6% of all mammary carcinomas and about 50% of all non-invasive cancers. Lobular carcinoma *in situ* is clinically silent and is usually an incidental finding in breast biopsies. It is not frequently associated with calcifications and, therefore, not diagnosed by mammography. It is commonly found exclusively in women in their fourth to fifth decade of life, predominantly in the premenopausal population.

LCIS has the propensity for multicentricity. Women with LCIS or LCIS with concurrent invasive carcinoma are at risk of having bilateral breast involvement in one-third and 60% of cases, respectively. When LCIS is diagnosed in the ipsilateral breast, about 40% of women will have disease in the contralateral breast as well. In addition, it is not uncommon to find LCIS as a companion lesion to intraductal carcinomas, sclerosing adenosis, fibroadenomas, radial scars and papillary hyperplasias.

Many consider LCIS as 'a marker lesion', which denotes increased risks for the development of subsequent invasive carcinoma, which is about 10 times that of the normal population. About a third of the lesions may actually progress to become invasive cancers.

The absolute risk for the development of invasive carcinoma is 20–25% at 15–20 years; and 15% in the contralateral breast after a diagnostic biopsy.

Histopathology The common histological appearance of LCIS consists of the total obliteration of the lobular lumina with malignant cells which are uniformly spaced and appear detached from each other. The nuclei are commonly hyperchromatic, centrally placed with small and discrete nucleoli and rare mitosis.

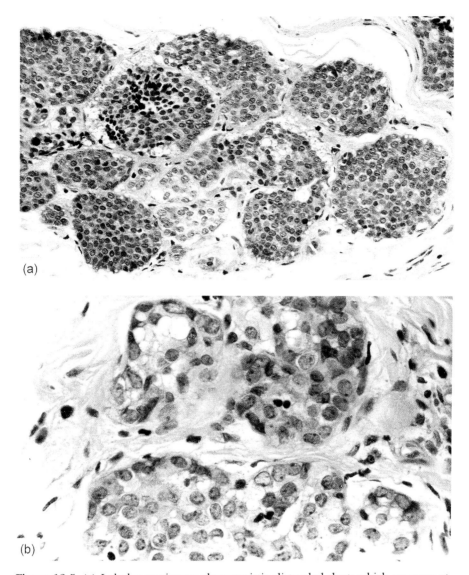

Figure 12.5 (a) Lobular carcinoma characteristic distended ducts which measure at least six cells in diameter (×200). Note the low nuclear grade. (b) At high magnification (×780) the cytoplasmic vacuolations are noted. Note absence of myoepithelial cell layer

The lobular glands are commonly distended; namely, the diameter will exceed six cells across (Figure 12.5). Myoepithelial cell layer may or may not be present. A commonly applied minimal diagnostic criterion of LCIS is when at least 50% of the glands within the lobule are involved. The glands proper should be totally filled by the malignant cells and some distinction of the glands should be present. An important characteristic of LCIS is the intracytoplasmic vacuolation of the cells which represents mucin, as confirmed by a histochemical stain such as mucicarmine (Figure 12.5b). Occasionally, increased cytoplasmic mucin content will displace the nucleus, yielding a signet cell appearance to the cell. Since mucin is absent from normal epithelia and myoepithelial cells, when present, it is an important diagnostic feature for LCIS. The disease originates, in pre-menopausal women, from the terminal duct lobular complex. However, in postmenopausal women where breast atrophy is present, LCIS originates from the terminal ducts. This is of significance, since in postmenopausal women duct involvement may be the only evidence for LCIS, appearing as a cloverleaf or as saw-toothed lumina. Commonly, the LCIS cells will infiltrate in-between normal duct cells, which will be displaced towards the lumen and the basally located myoepithelial cells.

For the pathologist, it is imperative to ensure that invasive disease is ruled out and that no malignant cells have violated the surrounding basement membrane. The invasion into the stroma by a few malignant cells can be subtle and deceiving. The presence of an inflammatory infiltrate and the desmoplastic reaction around LCIS should alert the pathologist to the possibility for invasive disease. The differential diagnosis consists primarily of proliferative lesions such as pseudolactational hyperplasia, myoepithelial hyperplasia, clear cell changes, and atypical lobular hyperplasia.

Prognosis LCIS is regarded by many as a 'marker' lesion for increased risk for the sub-sequent development of invasive carcinoma. The majority of patients treated by lumpec-tomy alone fare well. Several studies have shown that approximately 20–25% of the patients with LCIS will eventually develop car-cinoma in the ipsilateral breast and approxi-mately 10% in the contralateral breast. The majority of the patients with LCIS that develop carcinomas are of the invasive ductal type. Only 25% of the patients with LCIS will develop invasive lobular carcinomas.

Atypical lobular hyperplasia

Similar to atypical intraductal hyperplasia, the diagnostic criteria for atypical lobular hyper-plasia are subjective and not rigidly defined. Frequently, both quantitative and qualitative criteria are used jointly to render the correct diagnosis (Figure 12.6).

The minimal diagnostic criteria for atypical lobular hyperplasia consist of the presence of a diagnostic LCIS cell which involves the lobule only partially (less than 50%), without expanding glands, resulting in a lobule with indistinct borders between acinar units and intra-lobular ducts, in contrast to LCIS, where signifi-cant distension of acini is present.

Prognosis The presence of atypical lobular hyperplasia increases the risk for subsequent development of carcinoma. The risk increases with the duration of the follow-up and it ranges from 1.5 to 6 times that of the normal popula-tion. There are no additional risk factors in developing carcinoma in women with or with-out familial risk factors.

Infiltrative carcinomas of the breast

Invasive ductal carcinoma

Epidemiology and clinical presentation Invasive ductal carcinoma is predominantly a palpable solitary mass, frequently found in peri-meno-pausal woman in the sixth decade of life. This lesion represents approximately 75% of all inva-sive carcinomas of the breast. The precise origin of these lesions cannot be determined with cer-tainty. Hence, these have been lumped into a category defined as 'infiltrating ductal carci-noma' or 'adenocarcinoma of the breast, NOS.'

These tumors may contain some of the char-acteristics of the various tumors of the breast. Approximately 50% of all of these tumors are mixed with other types. For example, it is quite common to find isolated areas of the DCIS, lobular carcinoma, or other differentiated fea-tures in the midst of an infiltrating ductal carci-noma. It is difficult, if not impossible, to trace precisely the origin of infiltrating ductal carci-noma. The most common origin attributed to this poorly differentiated lesion is DCIS of the comedo type, while the better differentiated ones are thought to originate from the intraduc-tal cribriform variant.

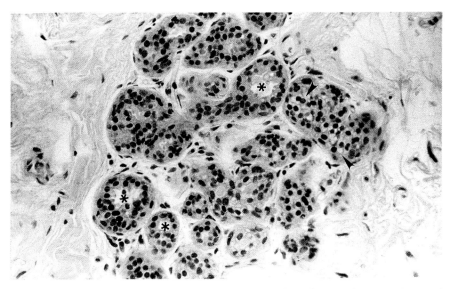

Figure 12.6 Atypical lobular hyperplasia. Minimal (less than 50%) expansion and distentions of lobules are present. Some luminal spaces are still preserved (asterisks), some cellular vacuolations and discohesiveness are noted (arrowheads) in the affected lobules

The histological grading of infiltrating ductal carcinoma, as with DCIS discussed earlier, is an attempt to correlate morphological parameters with clinical outcomes. The Scarf–Bloom–Richardson (SBR) grading method and its various modifications have evolved into a relatively accepted numerical scoring system of these lesions. It has been repeatedly shown that patients with lesions of high SBR scores have frequent lymph node involvement. This scoring method consists of grading three morphological parameters, each on a scale of 1–3. The maximum score of 9, calculated by adding individual grades of each of the categories, implies the poorest clinical (prognosis) behavior, while a score of 3 reflects a relatively well differentiated tumor.

The categories evaluated are gland or tubular formation – a reflection of differentiation, mitotic rate and nuclear morphology. As in the case of grading DCIS, the precise contribution of each of the components to the SBR score is uncertain, although several studies seem to indicate that nuclear grading is of greatest importance. However, histological grading must be considered together with tumor size,

circumscription of the lesion, vascular involvement, estrogen/progesterone-receptor (ER/PR) status, lymph node involvement, and others. A complete discussion reviewing prognostic factors in breast carcinoma is presented in Chapter 19.

Clinical presentation There are no unique features of infiltrating ductal carcinomas that would distinguish it from other palpable tumors of the breast.

Histological presentation On gross inspection, the cut surface of the tumor consists frequently of a stellate lesion, yellow-tan in color with chalky streaks radiating into the adjoining parenchyma. Microscopically, the tumor is heterogeneous. It may consist of nests or cords of cells dissecting through collagenized stroma or a group of cells attempting to form primitive gland-like structures (Figure 12.7a–c). Necrosis and calcifications may be present.

Inflammatory carcinoma is defined clinically as an erythematous skin lesion, warm to touch, with a peau d'orange texture with or without an underlying palpable mass. Microscopically, this

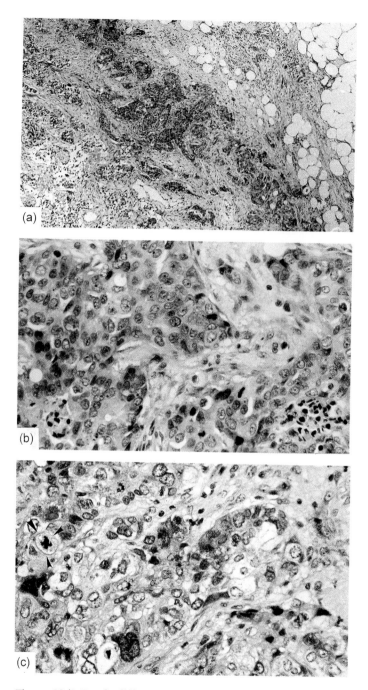

Figure 12.7 Poorly differentiated infiltrating ductal carcinoma is seen at low magnification. (a) Note the invasion of clusters of malignant cells throughout the breast stroma (×66). At high magnification (×330), (b) and (c), the intermediate (grade 2) and high grade (grade 3) nucleoli are noted. Note bizarre mitotic division in upper left corner (pointers)

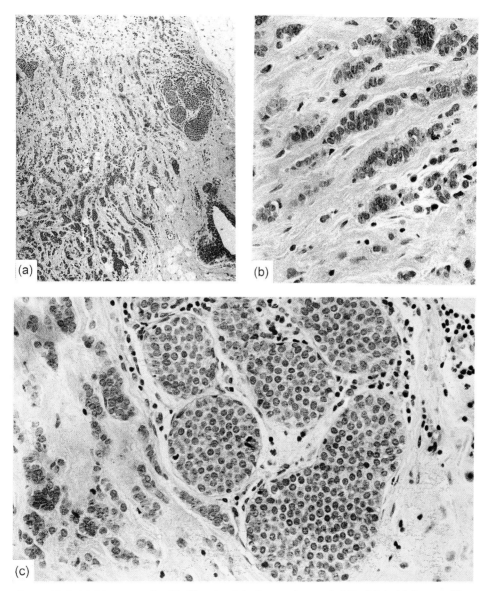

Figure 12.8 (a) Linear cords of infiltrating lobular carcinoma (×84). (b) At high magnifications, the infiltrating cells dissect through the stroma forming the characteristic 'Indian file' configuration (×420). (c) In the midst of infiltrating lobular carcinoma, a focus of lobular carcinoma *in situ* is present (×420)

entity consists of poorly differentiated infiltrating ductal carcinoma cells involving the dermal lymphatics, but frequently not involving the epidermis proper. It is noteworthy that despite a classical presentation of inflammatory carcinomas, as much as 50% of the patients may have a negative skin biopsy. The actual actuarial survival of infiltrating ductal carcinoma is 60% at 5 years and 47% at 10 years.

As a subset of infiltrating carcinomas, the concept of minimally invasive carcinoma was defined as those tumors with an aggregate of

<1 cm in diameter. Survival and recurrence rates in patients with minimal invasive carcinoma are better than that in patients with similar tumors of >1 cm in their largest dimension.

Infiltrating lobular carcinoma

Epidemiology and clinical presentation Invasive lobular carcinoma accounts for approximately up to 5% of all invasive cancers. The median age of patients is in the fifth decade of life with a broad range distribution from the second to the eighth decade, with somewhat higher frequency in older women. This tumor has a high propensity for bilaterality, reported to be as high as 40%.

The common clinical presentation is that of a skin-thickening or poorly defined palpable mass. Since calcifications are not common in infiltrating lobular carcinoma, false-negative mammographic studies are not uncommon.

Histopathology Frequently, the characteristic pattern of infiltrating lobular carcinoma is that of linear cords of cells, two cells wide, dubbed as 'Indian files', dissecting throughout the stroma (Figure 12.8a–c). In addition, such single files of cells may surround terminal ductules to form the classical 'targetoid pattern'. Other architectural variants have been described, such as the alveolar, solid and mixed pattern. The alveolar pattern consists of small discrete nests of cells, containing 20–40 cells each, separated by stroma. Cytologically, the cells are small, monomorphic at times, with intracellular lumina and containing mucin similar to those noted in lobular carcinoma *in situ*.

Prognosis Frequently, infiltrating lobular carcinomas involve lymph nodes in an insidious manner. The cellular infiltration is restricted primarily to the subcapsular and sinusoidal regions of the lymph nodes. Metastases to bone marrow are quite common and may go undetected to the untrained eye. Similarly, carcinomatosis, skeletal, retroperitoneal, and vertebral involvement occurs. Commonly,

ovarian and uterine metastases occur as well. The actual survival of infiltrating lobular carcinoma is similar to that of the infiltrating ductal carcinoma.

Tubular carcinoma

Epidemiology and clinical presentation Tubular carcinoma, originally thought to be an uncommon lesion, is being detected by mammography with greater frequency, especially when the lesions are less than 1 cm in diameter. Calcifications are noted frequently, but these are located within companion lesions and not the tubular carcinoma proper. A recent report identified that 9% of all lesions less than 1 cm in diameter represent tubular carcinomas. These lesions occur within the same age range as invasive lobular carcinomas, but are more prevalent in the latter half of the fifth decade of life.

Clinically, the lesion is detected as a recent onset palpable mass. Fixation to skin and retraction may occur. The lesion is predominantly found in a distal location, but occasionally central lactiferous ducts can be involved.

Histopathology Tubular carcinomas are characterized by small angulated glands, one cell thick with open lumina which simulate ductules and, hence, a 'well-differentiated' architecture (Figure 12.9). However, these glands have irregular contours devoid of a myoepithelial cell layer or basement membranes and may be haphazardly distributed throughout the stroma. Cytologically, the cells of tubular carcinomas are homogeneous with hyperchromatic nuclei without visible nucleoli. Mitoses are rare.

A common companion lesion to tubular carcinomas is intraductal carcinoma and, hence, the frequency of calcifications present on mammography. These are confined mostly to the non-tubular component. Similarly, *in situ* lobular carcinomas or atypical lobular hyperplasias are commonly associated with tubular carcinoma.

Prognosis Tubular carcinomas rarely metastasize and are considered to have a favorable

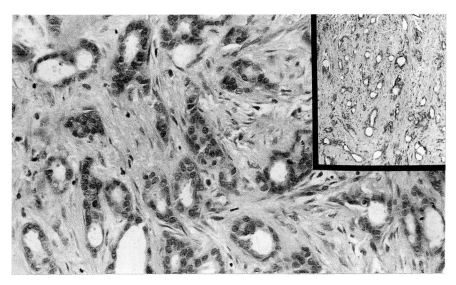

Figure 12.9 Infiltrating tubular carcinoma (inset ×78). At high magnification (×780), the malignant cells are organized as angulated glands with irregular outlines and devoid of myoepithelial cells. Note the low nuclear grade of these cells

prognosis. Only about 10% of patients with pure tubular carcinomas will develop lymph node metastasis, with a recurrence rate of less than 4% post-surgery. In contra-distinction, patients with tubulo–lobular variant experience a 30% actual lymph node involvement.

Medullary carcinoma

Epidemiology and clinical presentation Medullary carcinomas represent less than 10% of malignant breast tumors. Some epidemiological data suggest that there is a skewed racial distribution with a high prevalence among blacks. The mean age is between the mid-fourth to the mid-fifth decade. Clinically, the tumor is a well circumscribed, firm, palpable lesion. Bilaterality and multi-centricity of this lesion was reported. Not infrequently, nodes may be palpable secondary to a reactive process elicited by the tumor rather than true lymph node metastases.

Gross morphology and histological presentation Medullary carcinoma may be large bulky tumors with pushing borders, thus yielding the appearance of a lesion with well demarcated margins. Hemorrhage, necrosis, and cyst formations are frequently seen. Histologically, these tumors consist of large pleomorphic cells exhibiting a syncytial growth pattern, with abundant basophilic cytoplasm and nuclei with prominent nucleoli. Heterochromatin is prominent. Although these tumors bear morphological characteristics of high-grade, poorly differentiated lesions, histological grading criteria should not be applied. In general, these tumors have a very good prognosis if they meet the strict diagnostic criteria of medullary carcinoma. Medullary carcinomas must meet the following histological criteria to warrant this diagnosis:

1. Growth pattern.
2. High grade nuclei.
3. High mitotic rate.
4. Marked to intense lymphoplasmacytic infiltrate.

If the tumors do not have all these features, then the diagnosis of atypical medullary carcinoma should be rendered (Figure 12.10). It is important to make this distinction since atypical

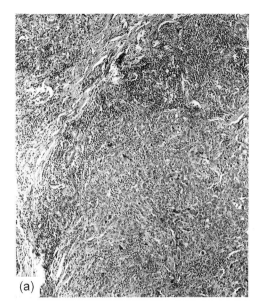
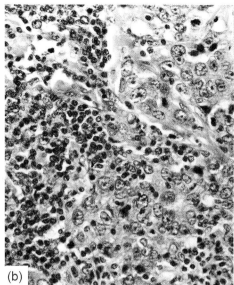

Figure 12.10 (a) Characteristic medullary carcinoma with a prominent pushing border consisting of solid sheets of cells and accompanying lymphocytic infiltrates (×78). (b) The lymphocytic infiltrate is present in the midst of malignant cells with high nuclear grade (×780)

medullary carcinoma has a poorer prognosis than medullary carcinoma (see below). Fifty per cent of these tumors are associated with intraductal carcinoma which is frequently found at the periphery of the tumor. Metaplastic reactions may be seen primarily of the squamous and mesenchymal type. Most medullary carcinomas have aneuploid DNA and are ER/PR negative.

Prognosis Patients with typical medullary carcinoma have a more favorable prognosis than patients with infiltrating ductal carcinomas. They have less lymph node involvement, although a higher false-positive rate on lymph node dissection is present. This is attributed to the intense reactivity of the lymph to the lymphohistiocytic infiltrate present in the classical medullary carcinoma.

Patients with tumors 3 cm in size or less have a better prognosis than those with larger tumors. Such patients with typical medullary carcinoma have a 90% chance of disease-free survival at 10 years. However, patients with lesions larger than 3 cm and lymph node involvement have a similar prognosis to patients with infiltrating carcinoma.

Patients with atypical medullary carcinomas, namely, those lesions which contain more than 25% non-syncytial patterns and tubuloglandular components, have a worse prognosis than the typical medullary carcinoma and it is similar to that of infiltrating ductal carcinoma.

Mucinous carcinoma

Epidemiology and clinical presentation Mucinous carcinomas account for 2% of all breast carcinomas. This malignancy occurs in all ages with a preponderance in older women. Clinically, these are palpable lesions which may or may not be fixed to the chest wall. Recently, smaller non-palpable mucinous carcinomas have been reported in younger women.

Gross and histopathological presentation The mucinous carcinomas are characterized as soft lesions containing large amounts of mucin which confer a glistening gelatinous consistency on gross inspection. The firmness of the lesion is determined by the amount of fibrous

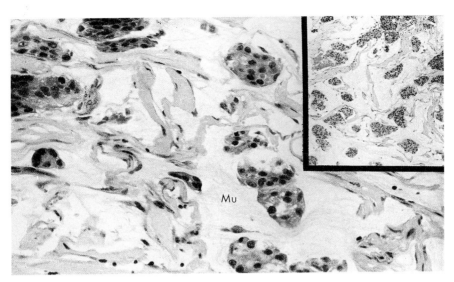

Figure 12.11 Mucinous carcinoma showing clusters of malignant cells dispersed in pools of mucin (Mu). Magnification ×780 (inset ×78)

tissue present. Microscopically, the malignant cells appear immersed in pools of mucin. This characteristic pattern must be present in most sections to establish the correct diagnosis (Figure 12.11). The criteria for the diagnosis of mucinous carcinoma are somewhat variable. Some investigators suggested that at least 50% of the lesion should consist of extracellular mucin. In about 75% of mucinous carcinomas, some intraductal carcinoma may be present. These were defined by Norris *et al.* as the 'mixed variant of mucinous carcinoma'. Since there are significant prognostic differences between pure and mixed mucinous carcinomas, this diagnostic distinction must be adhered to.

The majority of mucinous carcinomas are ER positive. Some histochemical and ultrastructural studies suggested a neuroendocrine origin of this tumor. In about 50% of tumors, argyrophilic granules are present. Tavasolli reported that these lesions are also S-100 positive. Rosen has suggested that the presence or absence of argyrophilic granules is of no prognostic significance.

Prognosis Pure mucinous carcinomas have a favorable prognosis when compared to infiltrating ductal carcinomas. Most patients do not develop lymph node metastasis. On the other hand, there is a higher incidence of lymph node involvement in patients with mixed mucinous carcinomas. Five-year survival post-treatment in pure mucinous carcinoma is approximately 90%, and 85% after 15 years post-mastectomy, while those with a mixed variant have a survival rate of only 60% at 15 years.

Paget's disease

Epidemiology and clinical presentation Paget's disease represents up to 5% of all breast carcinomas and may be found in females and males. As first described by Sir James Paget, this is an 'eczematous lesion' of the areolar and peri-areolar areas. Ulcerations of the skin may be present in the late stages of the disease. In approximately 50% of cases, a firm mass is palpable under the involved nipple/areolar complex (NAC) which may represent an underlying invasive carcinoma.

Histopathological features The diagnostic feature of this lesion is the presence of the so-called Paget's cells within the epithelium of the NAC. These are large cells with ample cytoplasm and large nuclei with prominent nucleoli

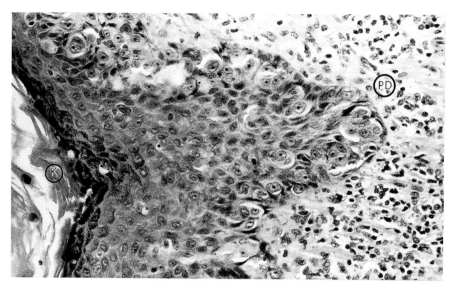

Figure 12.12 Paget's cells within the basal layer of the epidermis of the areola (×780). Paget's cells residing within the typical 'lacunae' or clear spaces with large nuclei and large nucleoli. Note intense lymphocytic infiltrate at the bottom right. K, keratin; PD, Paget's cells

(Figure 12.12). Immunohistochemically, these are CEA positive and may contain mucin, which may point to their lineage of mainly ductal cells. However, since these cells may contain melanin, they may be mistaken for malignant melanoma cells, a diagnosis which must be excluded.

These intra-epidermal malignant cells bear no relationship to the underlying invasive carcinoma when present. However, the absence of palpable mass does not exclude the presence of a non-invasive *in situ* carcinoma.

Prognosis When Paget's disease is not associated with an underlying carcinoma, surgical excision of the lesion is curative, with a 10-year survival rate of up to 100%. However, in the presence of an underlying carcinoma, the size of the lesion and lymph node status are important prognostic features. A palpable mass frequently represents an invasive carcinoma. The 5-year survival of such patients with lymph node involvement was reported as high as 70%. In patients without a palpable mass, the 5-year survival was 99%. Lymph node involvement, as predicted, results in a significant reduction in the 5-year survival rates.

Mesenchymal lesions Mesenchymal lesions of the breast are uncommon and bear similarity to soft tissue sarcomas of other anatomical sites. They originate from the breast stroma and may be regarded as non-epithelial malignancies of the breast. Included in this category are mammary sarcomas, malignant fibrohistiocytomas (MFH), leiomyosarcomas and angiosarcomas. Since some of these lesions are exceedingly rare (less than 1% of invasive carcinomas of the breast), their review is beyond the scope of this chapter. The interested reader should consult some of the recommended references at the end of this chapter.

An additional lesion which contains elements of both periductal and intralobular stroma is cystosarcoma phylloide (CP). This tumor belongs to a group of biphasic tumors characterized clinically by a course which cannot be predicated on histology alone. In malignant CP, the spindly stromal elements predominate, yielding a histology with features similar to soft tissue sarcoma.

Lymphomas of the breast are considered within the mesenchymal tumor group. These may be primary or secondary to systemic disease. Primary lymphoma of the breast is a rare tumor. It represents approximately 2% of all extranodal lymphomas and less than 1% of all breast malignancies.

Most primary lymphomas of the breast are diffuse large cell lymphomas, B-cell type. The cell of the origin is most likely the breast lymphocyte which is a part of the systemic mucosal immune system, such as MALT. Recently an increasing number of MALT lesions have been reported. The prognosis of breast lymphoma, with respect to recurrence and survival, is equal to that of other extra-nodal lymphomas and depends primarily on histological grade.

Bibliography

Bland, KJ, Copeland EM (eds). *The Breast – Comprehensive Management of Benign and Malignant Diseases*. Philadelphia: WB Saunders Co., 1991

Carter D. *Interpretation of Breast Biopsies*, 2nd edn. New York: Raven Press, 1990

Page D, Anderson TJ. *Diagnostic Histopathology of the Breast*. Edinburgh: Churchill Livingstone, 1987

Rosen PP. *Rosen's Breast Pathology*. Philadelphia: Lippincott-Raven, 1996

Silverstein MJ. *Ductal Carcinoma In Situ of the Breast*. Baltimore: Williams and Wilkins, 1997

Tavassoli FA. *Pathology of the Breast*. Norwalk: Appleton & Lange, 1992

Staging of breast cancer

13

L. Jardines and S.O. Asbell

The first staging system for breast cancer, the Columbia Clinical Classification, was developed by Dr Haagensen and was developed on the basis of his clinical experience between 1915 and 1942. The currently accepted system for breast cancer staging was developed by International Union Against Cancer (UICC) and the American Joint Commission on Cancer (AJCC). Staging can be accomplished by either clinical and radiological evaluation or after pathologic examination of a surgical specimen. The purpose of accurate staging is to determine the most appropriate form of therapy, determine prognosis and compare survival based upon different treatment regimens.

The AJCC/UICC staging system is based upon the evaluation of the tumor size (T), the nodal status (N) and distant metastatic disease (M) and is known as TNM. Clinical staging is notated as cTNM or TNM and pathologic staging is notated as pTNM.

Clinical staging includes the results of the physical examination, radiological studies and operative findings. Pathologic staging takes into account clinical factors and the results of pathologic evaluation of the operative specimen.

TNM NOMENCLATURE FOR BREAST CANCER

Clinical and pathologic staging of the tumor (T)

T_x	Primary tumor cannot be assessed
T_0	No evidence of primary tumor
T_{is}	Carcinoma *in situ*
T_1	≤2 cm
T_{1a}	≤0.5 cm
T_{1b}	0.5–1 cm
T_{1c}	>1–2 cm
T_2	>2–5 cm
T_3	>5 cm
T_4	Any size with direct extension to the chest wall or skin (excluding pectoral muscles)
T_{4a}	Extension to the chest wall
T_{4b}	Edema or ulceration of skin or presence of satellite nodules
T_{4c}	Both T_{4a} and T_{4b}
T_{4d}	Inflammatory carcinoma

Clinical staging of the axillary lymph nodes (N)

N_x	Regional nodes cannot be assessed
N_0	No nodal metastasis
N_1	Metastasis to movable ipsilateral axillary lymph node(s)
N_2	Metastasis to ipsilateral axillary lymph node(s) fixed to one another or to other structures
N_3	Metastasis to ipsilateral internal mammary lymph node(s)

Pathologic staging of the axillary lymph nodes

pNx	Regional lymph nodes cannot be assessed
pN0	Metastasis to one or more movable axillary nodes
pN1a	Micrometastasis only (none larger than 0.2 cm)

pN1   Metastasis to one or more movable lymph nodes

pN1b   Metastasis to one to more lymph nodes, any of which is larger than 0.2 cm in greatest dimension

pN1bi   Metastases, in one to three lymph nodes, any of which is larger than 0.2 cm in greatest dimension

pN1bii   Metastases to four or more lymph nodes, any of which is larger than 0.2 cm and all of which are less than 2 cm in greatest dimension

pN1biii   Extension of tumor beyond the capsule of a lymph node metastasis less than 2 cm in greatest dimension

pN2   Metastasis to ipsilateral nodes which are fixed to one another or other structures

pN3   Metastasis to one or more ipsilateral internal mammary lymph nodes

Metastasis (M)

M_x Presence of metastases cannot be assessed

M_0 No distant metastasis

M_1 Distant metastasis, including metastasis to supraclavicular lymph node(s)

Stages of primary breast cancer

	T	N	M
Stage 0	T_{is}	N_0	M_0
Stage I	T_1	N_0	M_0
Stage IIA	T_0	N_1	M_0
	T_1	N_1	M_0
	T_2	N_0	M_0
Stage IIB	T_2	N_1	M_0
	T_3	N_0	M_0
Stage IIIA	T_0	N_2	M_0
	T_1	N_2	M_0
	T_2	N_2	M_0
	T_3	N_1	M_0
	T_3	N_2	M_0
Stage IIIB	T_4	Any N	M_0
	Any T	N_3	M_0
Stage IV	Any T	Any N	Any M

PRETREATMENT STAGING EVALUATION FOR PATIENTS WITH BREAST CANCER

The optimal preoperative staging evaluation for patients with breast cancer has not been established and often varies from practitioner to practitioner. The author will provide her strategies in preoperative staging based upon the extent of locoregional disease. The studies performed are based upon tumor size, the clinical examination of the axilla, the presence of symptoms suggestive of metastatic disease and the likelihood of systemic metastases based upon the locoregional extent of disease.

Those patients with ductal carcinoma *in situ* require only a complete physical examination and bilateral mammography to evaluate the extent of the disease. Patients who present with a T_1 or small T_2 breast cancer, a clinically negative axilla and no complaints suggestive of distant metastases require bilateral mammography, chest radiography and liver function tests as their initial preoperative staging evaluation. If the mammogram does not reveal any new findings and the remainder of the studies are normal, no additional evaluation is necessary prior to beginning therapy. Some practitioners always obtain a baseline bone scan no matter what the clinical stage of disease to serve as a comparative study should the patient develop bone complaints or an elevated alkaline phosphatase in the future; however, this is not cost-effective. When a patient is found to have abnormal liver function tests and/or an abnormality on chest radiography, metastatic disease must be excluded prior to beginning therapy.

Those patients with large T_2 lesions as well as T_3 or T_4 tumors with or without a clinically positive axilla on presentation require a thorough pretreatment evaluation to exclude distant metastatic disease. Patients should undergo bilateral mammography, chest radiography, a radionuclide bone scan and computed tomography (CT) of the liver with intravenous contrast to evaluate completely the extent of disease. In patients who have a contraindication to intravenous contrast, magnetic resonance imaging of the liver can be substituted for the CT scan. Magnetic resonance imaging or computed tomography of the brain and spine are not routinely performed and are indicated only if the patient is symptomatic.

Bibliography

American Joint Committee on Cancer Staging and End Results Reporting. In Beahrs OH, Henson DE, Hutter RVP *et al.*, eds. *Manual for Staging of Cancer*, 4th edn. Philadelphia, JB Lippincott, 1992:149

Haagensen CD, Stout AP. Carcinoma of the breast. Criteria for operability. *Ann Surg* 1943;118:859–70

NCCN Breast Cancer Practice Guidelines. *Oncology* 1996;10 (supplement): 47–75

Surgical management of breast cancer

14

L. Jardines

NON-INVASIVE BREAST CANCER

Lobular carcinoma *in situ*

The term lobular carcinoma *in situ* (LCIS) was coined by Foote and Stewart in 1941 and described a form of *in situ* breast cancer which developed from the terminal lobules. Initially, LCIS was treated by radical surgery; however, the current feeling is that LCIS is more of a marker for increased breast cancer risk. Therefore, it has been suggested by breast pathologists that a more appropriate term for this pathologic entity may be lobular neoplasia.

Incidence

LCIS affects only women, has a peak incidence at age 45 and decreases in incidence after menopause. Up to 90% of women diagnosed with LCIS are premenopausal whereas only 30% of women with invasive breast cancer are in this category. LCIS is found more frequently in Caucasian women when compared to African–American women in the United States. Interestingly, most cases of LCIS are hormone receptor positive. Therefore, there may be hormonal influences related to the development of LCIS.

In the literature, the incidence of LCIS has ranged from 0.5 to 3.6% in breast biopsy specimens; however, the true incidence of LCIS is unknown since the disease is non-palpable and there are no radiologic findings associated with it. With a breast biopsy, different amounts of normal breast tissue may be removed and subsequently analyzed. LCIS is most often identified as an incidental finding when a breast biopsy has been performed for another reason. The apparent incidence is increasing as more breast biopsies are performed, pathologists are examining the specimen more thoroughly and LCIS is being recognized as a pathologic entity to a greater degree. This entity is often bilateral and multicentric. Based upon data from mastectomy specimens, LCIS was found to be multifocal in 60–80% of cases. Patients with LCIS had previously undergone mirror image biopsy of the contralateral breast and 23–35% were found to have LCIS bilaterally. The presence of bilateral LCIS does not increase the breast cancer risk (Table 14.1).

Natural history

There have been several long-term studies of women who had been diagnosed with LCIS and treated with biopsy alone to determine their risk of developing an invasive breast cancer. The follow-up in these studies ranges from 5 to 24 years and breast cancer developed in 6.3–34.5%. In the largest series by Haagensen

Table 14.1 Characteristics of LCIS

- Bilateral
- Multicentric
- Found only in women
- Non-palpable
- Diagnosed incidentally

with 287 patients and 16.3 years of follow-up, 18% of the patients developed an invasive breast cancer. The relative risk is 7–12 for developing an invasive breast cancer after the diagnosis of LCIS is made. The absolute risk for the development of an invasive breast cancer is 20–25%. The risk for developing an invasive breast cancer may be greatest during the first 15 years after the diagnosis is made and then drop off subsequently.

Several studies demonstrated that the invasive breast cancer has approximately an equal chance of developing in either breast. The majority of patients who develop invasive carcinoma of the breast after LCIS are found to have invasive ductal carcinoma. In the literature, infiltrating lobular carcinoma was diagnosed in 25–36% of cases where the patient had a previous diagnosis of LCIS. Overall, infiltrating lobular carcinoma comprises approximately 5–10% of all breast cancers; therefore, the incidence of this histology is found with a greater frequency in women with a prior history of LCIS.

Treatment (Table 14.2)

Patients with LCIS are at high risk to develop breast cancer; however, most women who have a diagnosis of LCIS do not develop invasive breast carcinoma. After the diagnosis has been established by biopsy, there is no need to re-excise the areas to obtain negative surgical margins. In addition, there is no need for chemotherapy or breast irradiation. A reasonable and frequently chosen option for their management is close follow-up with annual mammography and clinical breast examination at 4- to 6-month intervals. Patients who choose this option are followed for the remainder of their lives, since the risk for developing an invasive cancer is approximately 1% per year.

Some patients are uncomfortable with close follow-up and may choose prophylactic bilateral total mastectomies with the option of immediate reconstruction. Some surgeons have utilized a subcutaneous mastectomy where the incision is

Table 14.2 Treatment of LCIS

- Close observation
- Bilateral mastectomies with immediate reconstruction
- Participation in a chemoprevention trial

placed in the inframammary fold, the nipple–areolar complex is spared and an implant can be placed to reconstruct the breast mound. It has been estimated that 5–10% of the breast tissue is not excised after subcutaneous mastectomy due to the location of the incision and the retention of the nipple–areolar complex. In the case of prophylactic subcutaneous mastectomy, there are no data to suggest that breast cancer risk can be reduced in high risk women by reducing the volume of breast tissue. Breast cancer has developed in women who have undergone this type of surgery and women who have been treated in this way may have a false sense of security.

With total mastectomy, a small ellipse of skin is excised around the nipple–areolar complex. Due to the location of the incision, there is better visualization to dissect the skin flaps. In addition, the nipple–areolar complex is resected. Therefore, less breast tissue remains on the chest wall after this procedure when compared to a subcutaneous mastectomy. There are no studies to date which analyze the reduction in breast cancer risk after prophylactic mastectomy and there are reports in the literature of breast cancer developing after prophylactic total mastectomy. The use of unilateral mastectomy with mirror image biopsy is not recommended, since each breast is at risk and most patients with LCIS do not develop invasive breast cancer.

Women with LCIS may also consider participating in a chemoprevention study. The National Surgical Adjuvant Breast and Bowel Project (NSABP) recently released preliminary data on their chemoprevention study where tamoxifen was used as the chemopreventative agent. Tamoxifen, an anti-estrogen, had been used as adjuvant treatment for women with breast cancer. When the studies were analyzed, it was found that tamoxifen could reduce the incidence of a contralateral breast cancer by approximately 40%. This raised the question as to whether tamoxifen could prevent breast cancer in high-risk women. The NSABP P-01 trial was a prospective randomized trial where patients at high risk for breast cancer were randomized to receive either tamoxifen or placebo for 5 years. Early analysis revealed a ≥45% reduction in breast cancer incidence in a high risk population.

Ductal carcinoma *in situ*

Ductal carcinoma *in situ* (DCIS) is being encountered more frequently with the expanded use of screening mammography. In some institutions, DCIS accounts for 25–50% of all breast cancers. It occurs more frequently and is more likely to progress to invasive disease than LCIS. DCIS, like invasive ductal carcinoma, occurs more frequently in women, although it accounts for approximately 5% of all male breast cancers. The average age at diagnosis is 54–56 years, which is approximately a decade later than the age at presentation for LCIS. The risk of developing an invasive carcinoma following a biopsy diagnosis of DCIS is between 25 and 50%. Virtually all invasive cancers which follow DCIS are ductal, ipsilateral and generally present within 10 years of diagnosing the DCIS within the same quadrant of the breast. It is for these reasons that DCIS is a more ominous lesion and appears to be a more direct precursor of invasive cancer. The disease is less commonly bilateral when compared to LCIS and there is approximately a 30% incidence of multicentricity. The clinical signs of DCIS include a mass, breast pain or bloody nipple discharge; however, the disease most often presents as microcalcifications on mammography (Table 14.3).

Different histologic subtypes of DCIS have been described and include papillary, solid, cribriform and comedo. Some breast pathologists simply divide DCIS into non-comedo and comedo. The comedo variant of DCIS has been associated with a more aggressive behavior, with increased incidence of ipsilateral breast tumor recurrence and foci of microinvasion. Overexpression of oncogenes, loss of tumor suppresser genes and aneuploidy have been seen to a greater degree in comedo DCIS, which may be responsible for its aggressive behavior.

The treatment for DCIS is evolving and in the past, mastectomy has been the standard treatment (Table 14.4). Following mastectomy for DCIS, the recurrence rate is approximately 1% and the overall survival rate is 98–99% at 10 years. In more recent times, less radical surgery in combination with adjuvant breast irradiation has been utilized with the overall survival equal to that of mastectomy when there are no contraindications to breast conservation. The incidence of positive lymph nodes after axillary dissection for DCIS is only 1–2% and therefore, generally, resection is not indicated.

Some patients with smaller tumors have been treated with lumpectomy with or without adjuvant breast irradiation. As with invasive breast cancer, the surgical margins should be free of tumor. If the DCIS is diagnosed by microcalcifications on mammography, the patient should have a post-biopsy mammogram to ensure that all of the microcalcifications have been excised. If the post-biopsy mammogram is positive, the patient should undergo re-excision under needle localization guidance.

Table 14.3 Characteristics of DCIS

- Unilateral, generally
- Unifocal, generally
- Found in women and men
- Diagnosed on mammography and/or physical examination

Table 14.4 Treatment of DCIS

- Lumpectomy with or without adjuvant breast irradiation
- Total mastectomy
- Axillary lymph node dissection generally not indicated

The NSABP B-17 trial was a prospective randomized trial in which patients with DCIS were treated with lumpectomy and had pathologic confirmation of negative surgical margins. Patients were then randomized to receive no further therapy or adjuvant breast irradiation. From their data, adjuvant breast irradiation appears to be beneficial in preventing a local breast recurrence after lumpectomy, by approximately 50%. In addition, they observed that those patients treated with lumpectomy and radiation who developed an ipsilateral breast tumor recurrence were more likely to have non-invasive disease. On the other hand, patients who were treated with lumpectomy alone and developed a recurrence were more likely to have invasive disease. The local failure rate after wide excision alone for DCIS varies from 10 to 63%, whereas the local failure rate following wide excision and radiation therapy is significantly lower and ranges from 7 to 21%. There may be a population of patients where wide excision alone is appropriate and this would include patients with small tumors (<0.5–1 cm) which are subclinical and have favorable histologies (non-comedo).

If a patient develops a local failure after conservative surgery and radiation therapy for DCIS, it is generally in the region of the initial primary tumor. The treatment of an ipsilateral breast tumor recurrence after conservative treatment for DCIS where there is no evidence of distant metastatic disease is mastectomy.

The optimal treatment for DCIS has yet to be determined and continues to evolve.

STAGE I–II INVASIVE BREAST CANCER

The treatment of early stage invasive breast cancer, stage I–II, continues to evolve. Modified radical mastectomy remains the most common form of surgical therapy for breast cancer in the United States and there are very few indications for radical mastectomy. Breast conservation therapy combines lumpectomy or partial mastectomy with adjuvant breast irradiation.

The idea of breast conservation therapy is not new, but has become an accepted alternative to mastectomy based upon the results of numerous prospective and retrospective studies. The National Surgical Adjuvant Breast and Bowel Project (NSABP) in the United States and other groups in Europe developed clinical trials to determine whether breast conservation could play a role in the treatment of breast cancer. The NSABP compared mastectomy to lumpectomy and axillary lymph node dissection with or without adjuvant breast irradiation in the B-06 trial and found that the overall survival in all of the groups was essentially the same. The disease-free survival in the group of patients treated by lumpectomy and axillary dissection without breast irradiation was considerably shorter than that observed for patients in the other treatment arms. The study demonstrated that lumpectomy, axillary lymph node dissection along with breast irradiation was equal to modified radical mastectomy in both disease-free survival and overall survival when patients were properly selected. In addition, this trial demonstrated the importance of adjuvant breast irradiation in reducing local breast recurrence. These results have been reproduced in many other prospective randomized clinical trials as well as retrospective studies, and since the mid-1980s thousands of patients have been treated with breast-conserving treatment in the United States and Europe.

In the United States, there are regional variations in the rates at which breast conservation is performed. In the Northeast, patients are more likely to undergo breast conserving treatment, while in the South they are more likely to undergo mastectomy.

Patient selection

There are specific guidelines which must be followed when selecting patients for breast conservation therapy. First, the patients should be motivated for breast conservation therapy since it entails daily travel to the radiation therapy facility. There are other patients who are not considered candidates for conservative surgery and radiation either because the risk of recurrence following the conservative approach is significant enough to warrant mastectomy, or because the likelihood of an unacceptable cosmetic result is high.

Patients who are being considered for breast conservation should undergo a careful history and physical examination. If the tumor is palpable, the size, location and mobility within the breast should be assessed. Bilateral mammography should be obtained to determine whether there are other sites of disease within the ipsilateral breast and to survey the contralateral breast. If the tumor is palpable, fine needle aspiration cytology can be performed to facilitate discussions with the patient concerning treatment options. It is best if the patient and her family can meet with a multispecialty group consisting of a surgeon, radiation oncologist, medical oncologist and plastic surgeon so that she can make an informed decision concerning her care. If the patient desires breast conservation therapy, the initial breast surgery should be a lumpectomy or partial mastectomy where the tumor is removed with a margin of normal breast tissue. The specimen should be marked with suture in the operating room to provide orientation prior to sending it to pathology. The pathologist should ink the specimen to facilitate the evaluation of the surgical resection margins.

There are a number of considerations in the decision-making process concerning appropriate local/regional treatment for early breast cancer, which include primary tumor size and location, the overall breast size or total body weight, and a history of pre-existing collagen vascular disease (Table 14.5). Patients with multicentric breast cancer diagnosed either by biopsy or by mammography (diffuse microcalcifications) are not candidates for breast conservation since there is a high likelihood of the patient having a significant amount of residual disease within the breast after the initial surgical treatment. This condition has been associated with a high risk of breast recurrence. When the tumor is greater than 4–5 cm, the patient is generally

Table 14.5 Considerations for breast conservation therapy

- Patient motivation
- Tumor size
- Breast size
- Multicentric disease
- Tumor location
- Collagen–vascular disease
- Prior radiation
- Margin status
- Pregnancy
- Extensive intraductal component
- Tumor histology

not considered a candidate for breast conservation due to the risk of significant residual tumor burden following lumpectomy and the likelihood of a poor cosmetic result following lumpectomy. Patients with centrally located tumors requiring excision of the nipple–areolar complex traditionally have not been offered breast conservation; however, the cosmetic result obtained after local excision of the tumor which includes the nipple–areolar complex may not be much different from that obtained following mastectomy and reconstruction. In addition, the surgical procedure is less extensive and the patient has a sensate breast and chest wall when compared to mastectomy and immediate reconstruction. Recent studies also indicate that patients with centrally located primary tumors can be safely treated by the conservative approach. Patients who present with nipple discharge related to an underlying breast carcinoma may not be candidates for breast conservation, since this presentation has been associated with a high local failure rate. Individuals treated with prior irradiation to the breast region, such as mantle irradiation for Hodgkin's disease, are not candidates for breast conservation therapy and should be treated with mastectomy. Pregnancy is a relative contraindication to breast conservation therapy, since it is extremely difficult to evaluate the breasts by mammography to determine whether the disease is multifocal. When breast conservation therapy is considered in the face of pregnancy the radiation therapy should be delayed until after delivery. In addition, there are no reports in the literature concerning local recurrence after breast conservation in the pregnant woman.

Other factors to consider take into account the risk for ipsilateral breast tumor recurrence. The available data suggest that the status of the surgical margins is important in assessing the risk of recurrence. When margins are negative or close, the risk of recurrence is extremely low; however, when margins are positive, the risk for local recurrence increases, as does the risk for systemic metastases. An extensive intraductal component (EIC) is defined as the simultaneous presence of an intraductal carcinoma comprising 25% or more of the primary invasive tumor and/or an intraductal carcinoma within the surrounding normal breast tissue. Initial studies suggested that the local recurrence rate after breast conservation therapy with an EIC positive tumor was high. Subsequent reports determined that patients with EIC positive tumors who have negative surgical margins can be successfully treated with breast conservation therapy. The association between hormone receptor status, patient age, the presence of lymphovascular invasion and histology on ipsilateral breast recurrence is less well defined. Young age is often defined as age less than 35 or 40 and numerous studies have evaluated the effects of young age on the incidence of local/regional recurrence following breast conservation therapy. In some reports, young patients have a higher incidence of local failure; however, this may be associated with a high incidence of other poor prognostic factors such as high histologic grade, tumor necrosis and lymphovascular permeation. In other studies, with adequate surgery, assessment of surgical margins and the use of adjuvant chemotherapy for node-positive patients, there is no increased risk of local/ regional recurrence in young patients. In other studies, young patients had a higher risk of local regional recurrence no matter whether they were treated with breast conservation therapy or mastectomy. The local recurrence rates for invasive lobular carcinoma have been reported as being greater than that

seen for invasive ductal carcinoma. In other studies, patients with invasive lobular carcinoma had similar recurrence rates when compared to patients with invasive ductal histology; therefore, patients with invasive lobular carcinoma should not be excluded from conservative treatment on the basis of histology. Lymphovascular permeation had been identified as a risk factor for local/regional recurrence; however, in multivariate analysis, it was not significant. In univariate analysis, estrogen receptor negativity was associated with an increased risk for local recurrence but was not a significant factor in multivariate analysis. The presence of histologically positive nodes is not a contraindication for breast conservation therapy.

Role of axillary lymph node dissection in invasive breast cancer

Approximately 70% of patients with invasive breast cancer present with stage I–II disease. Breast cancer metastasizes via lymphatics to regional nodes (axillary, supraclavicular or internal mammary) or hematogenously to distant sites. There have been a variety of factors which have been associated with axillary nodal metastases and include tumor size, location, clinical stage of disease and other tumor characteristics. The presence of tumor-containing lymph nodes as well as the absolute number of positive lymph nodes are important prognostic indicators and have been used to identify patients who are candidates for adjuvant chemotherapy, hormonal therapy and/or radiation therapy. Another reason proposed for the use of axillary lymph node dissection is to diminish the likelihood of regional recurrence, since many patients may have clinically occult disease and dissection of these involved nodes may prevent a relapse. There is controversy concerning the use of axillary dissection in all patients with breast cancer.

Axillary metastases

The most common initial site of spread of breast cancer is to the axillary lymph nodes, which probably results from tumor cell invasion into the lymphatic channels within the breast followed by spread to the axillary nodes secondary to the proximity of the tumor to the nodal basin. Lesions located in the upper outer quadrant of the breast are more likely to have associated lymph node metastases followed by retroareolar and lower outer quadrant lesions. It may be related to lymphatic drainage patterns, since lesions located in the inner quadrants are more likely to spread to the internal mammary nodes. A high percentage of patients with outer quadrant lesions will have axillary nodal disease regardless of tumor size.

The incidence of axillary nodal metastases has also been associated with the size of the primary tumor. Invasive tumors less than 1 cm have been associated with a 22% incidence of axillary disease. The incidence of axillary nodal metastases increases to approximately 50% with tumors up to 5–6 cm. In addition, the median number of positive lymph nodes in the axilla is proportional to the size of the tumor and range from two positive nodes for tumors less than 2 cm to six for lesions ranging from 5 to 7 cm.

Clinical stage is also an indicator for the likelihood of axillary metastases and as the stage increases so does the likelihood of axillary disease. Patients who are clinical stage I have an 18% chance of having disease identified in the axilla following dissection. For patients who are T_2N_0, there is a 30% chance of having occult axillary metastases. In patients who are clinical stage $T_{1,2}N_1$, the likelihood of identifying metastatic disease to the axillary nodes after dissection and pathologic review of the lymph nodes increases to 71%.

The status of the axillary lymph nodes may be evaluated either clinically or pathologically. It is clear that clinical examination is not as accurate as pathologic evaluation. If one compares the two methods at the same time, the false-negative and -positive rates can be determined. In eight series, the false-negative rate (clinically negative, pathologically positive) ranged from 21 to 39%, with a mean of 32.1%. The false-positive rate ranged from 7 to 55%,

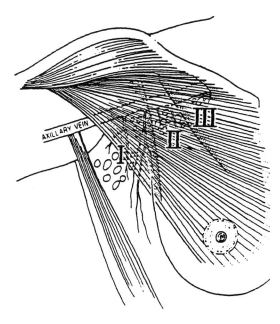

Figure 14.1 Axillary lymph node levels by level. Level I, low axilla, is lateral to the pectoralis minor muscle. Level II, mid-axilla, is posterior to the muscle. Level III, axillary apex, is lateral to the pectoralis minor muscle. Reproduced with permission from Harris JR, Morrow M. Treatment of early stage breast cancer. In Harris JR, Lipman ME, Morrow M, Hellman S, eds. *Diseases of the Breast*. Philadelphia: Lippincott-Raven, 1995:508

with a mean of 32.8%. For accurate staging of the patient, lymph node dissection is required. (It should be noted that the axilla should be clinically evaluated prior to breast biopsy, since it may be difficult to determine whether lymph node enlargement is on the basis of inflammatory changes secondary to surgery or to tumor.)

The distribution of nodal metastases within the axilla has also been studied by several groups. The levels of the axilla have been divided into three areas (Figure 14.1). The upper limit in all levels is the axillary vein. Level I is bounded by the medial border of the latissimus dorsi and the lateral border of the pectoralis minor muscle. Level II lies directly below the pectoralis minor muscle and level III extends from the lateral border of the pectoralis minor muscle to the subclavius muscle (Halstead's ligament). When axillary metastases are present, they most frequently involve level I. This is true whether level I nodes are involved alone or in combination with other nodes. The next most commonly involved is level II. It is possible to see nodal involvement of level II alone with the incidence ranging from 1.2 to 21.5% depending upon the series or level II–III involvement; however, this is less likely. When level III nodes are involved, it is most likely in conjunction with nodal metastases at other levels and it is rare to see nodal metastases to level III in the absence of disease at the two lower levels. With dissection of only level I (an axillary sampling), there is approximately a 25% chance of missing pathologically positive disease at higher levels (primarily level II).

Prognostic considerations of axillary lymph node dissection

Not only is the presence of disease in axillary lymph nodes important in prognosis for stage I–II breast cancer, but the number of involved nodes is also important in predicting outcome. The disease-free survival and overall survival is significantly better in node-negative patients when compared to those who are node-positive. In addition, survival decreases as the number of involved lymph nodes increase. In an early NSABP study, patients with one to three positive lymph nodes had a 35.5% disease-free survival and 37.5% overall survival at 10 years. In the same study, patients who had more than four positive lymph nodes had a 13.8% disease-free survival and a 13.4% overall survival over the same time interval. In addition, the number of involved lymph nodes has correlated with the likelihood for local/regional recurrence, and the likelihood of recurrence increases with the number of positive nodes.

Axillary recurrence in clinical node-negative patients treated by mastectomy alone

There are several series available where patients who were clinically node negative were treated by mastectomy alone. There are several clinical series where the follow-up extends to 10 years post-surgery and the incidence of axillary recurrence ranged from 16 to 37%. When all of the studies were analyzed, the average recurrence rate was 23.1%. When one compares this figure to the incidence of positive nodes in a clinically negative axilla (32.1%), there is the suggestion that a certain fraction of patients who have a clinically negative axilla have disease in the nodes, which when left alone does not become clinically apparent. Local recurrence in the axilla is less than 2% after axillary lymph node dissection where 10 or more nodes have been identified in the specimen.

Effect of axillary lymph node dissection on overall survival

An early study by the NSABP found that there was no improvement in overall survival when axillary lymph node dissection was included in the initial surgical therapy. It is important to keep in mind, however, that this is an early study and patients who participated in the trial were not treated with adjuvant systemic therapy, no matter what their nodal status was. Presently, recommendations for adjuvant therapy are based upon the presence or absence of positive nodes. In addition, if nodal disease is identified, the number of positive nodes can factor into which adjuvant therapy regimen is offered.

A recent report appeared in the literature suggesting that axillary lymph node dissection did improve survival in patients with early stage breast cancer. Patients with tumors less than 3 cm and clinically negative axillae were randomized to undergo lumpectomy + breast irradiation ± axillary lymph node dissection. Patients who were ER positive received adjuvant tamoxifen. The patients who underwent axillary lymph node dissection and were found to have metastatic disease received adjuvant chemotherapy. The patients treated with axillary lymph node dissection had an improved overall survival when compared to the group that did not. It is interesting to note, however, that there were 60 patients out of 326 in the axillary lymph node dissection arm who had positive lymph nodes and they were treated by systemic chemotherapy. Since the patients in each arm were similar, it is reasonable to assume that there were probably approximately the same number of patients with positive axillary nodes in the no-dissection arm who had occult axillary disease and received no systemic therapy. It seems that axillary lymph node dissection allows for more accurate staging and appropriate adjuvant treatment.

Considerations for the role of axillary lymph node dissection in breast cancer

Axillary lymph node dissection had been considered to be an absolute necessity as a part of the local treatment of breast cancer, whether the local surgical treatment was mastectomy or lumpectomy with adjuvant breast irradiation. The major role of axillary node dissection is to provide prognostic information which will guide further therapy. When axillary dissection is used in conjunction with lumpectomy and adjuvant radiation, it simplifies the radiation delivery to the breast. There has been an increased tendency to deliver adjuvant chemotherapy whether axillary nodes are involved or not; therefore, some have questioned whether lymph node dissection should be performed.

The morbidity related to axillary node dissection is generally low and is proportional to the extent of dissection. Major complications are extremely rare and include injury or thrombosis of the axillary vein and injury to the brachial plexus or motor nerves of the axilla. Minor complications are more common and include seroma formation, loss of sensation in the distribution of the intercostobrachial nerve, shoulder dysfunction, lymphedema of the arm or breast edema (in cases of breast preservation) and wound infection. Lymphedema is evaluated by measuring the circumference of the upper extremities 10 cm above and below the olecranon. The most common definition of lymphedema is an increase in circumference of 2 cm in the operated arm. The incidence of

postoperative lymphedema is reported to be as high as 15–20%; however, when a level I–II dissection is performed, the incidence of lymphedema is generally 3–5%.

Whether axillary lymph node dissection should be eliminated will depend upon the institutional approach towards the use of adjuvant therapy. Patients who would not otherwise be candidates for adjuvant treatment, such as women with invasive tumors <1 cm, should undergo axillary node dissection, since the identification of nodes with metastases would dramatically alter treatment. In addition, women participating in clinical trials which require complete staging should undergo axillary node dissection. The type of chemotherapy administered may differ depending on the extent of nodal involvement and an adriamycin containing regimen may be considered when there are four or more positive nodes. Furthermore, patients with 10 or more positive axillary nodes may be candidates to participate in bone marrow transplant/stem cell infusion trials. In a woman with a clinically negative axilla who is undergoing breast conservation where the results of the nodal dissection will not change the decisions concerning adjuvant treatment, consideration should be given to utilizing axillary irradiation in conjunction with breast irradiation to provide local control. In women who are being treated with mastectomy, axillary dissection should be incorporated into the surgical procedure.

Future considerations

The use of intraoperative vital dyes has been studied in patients with malignant melanoma. The technique was developed to identify patients with occult metastases to regional lymph nodes and who will benefit from lymph node dissection. A vital dye is injected in the region of the tumor, the dye-stained lymphatics are dissected and the first draining lymph node (the sentinel node) is excised and sent for evaluation. If positive, a lymph node dissection is performed. If negative, there is no further dissection.

Currently, studies are underway to determine if this technique is applicable to breast cancer.

Presently, all patients undergoing conservative therapy for invasive breast cancer receive adjuvant breast irradiation as part of the initial therapy. There are some data to suggest that patients whose tumors are less than 1 cm may not necessarily need breast irradiation as part of their therapy. However, until the data are available as a result of a prospective randomized trial, this modality is recommended as part of the initial therapy.

Surgical therapy for locally advanced breast cancer

Locally advanced breast cancers without evidence of distant metastases (stage IIIA and IIIB) account for approximately 20–25% of all breast cancers at presentation. The majority of locally advanced breast cancers are operable at presentation and can be surgically treated by mastectomy. Approximately 5–10% are inoperable secondary to tumor factors such as fixation to the chest wall, nodal factors which include the presence of matted nodes, or both. Between 66 and 90% of patients with stage III breast cancer will have lymph node involvement at the time of dissection, and approximately 50% will have four or more positive nodes.

The initial evaluation of a patient with a locally advanced breast cancer includes a thorough history and physical examination. On physical examination, if a mass is identified, it should be measured and the location within the breast should be documented. If the patient has inflammatory breast cancer, a mass within the breast is often not present but there is generally diffuse thickening of the breast parenchyma along with erythema and thickening of the skin. In addition, the patient should be examined carefully for skin nodules and ulceration as well as fixation of the tumor to the skin and/or underlying chest wall. The regional lymph node-bearing areas (supraclavicular, infraclavicular and axillary areas) should be examined. If supraclavicular or infraclavicular nodes are palpated, a fine needle aspiration should be performed, since disease in these areas would upstage the disease to stage IV. If nodes are detected in the ipsilateral axilla, the number, size and mobility should be assessed and documented. Routine laboratory studies should be performed and include liver function tests. A chest radiograph should be obtained to rule out metastatic disease to the lungs. Bilateral mammography should be performed to evaluate the extent of disease within the involved breast and to evaluate the contralateral breast. A bone scan and CT of the liver with intravenous contrast should also be performed to rule out other sites of metastatic disease.

The diagnosis of breast cancer may be established by fine needle aspiration, core biopsy or incisional biopsy. Hormone receptor status and flow studies can be performed on material obtained from a needle aspirate; however, it must be fixed properly. In some instances, i.e. a protocol, tissue must be obtained and this can be obtained through either a core or incisional biopsy.

A variety of treatment modalities have been used over the years for locally advanced breast cancer. The 5-year survival for patients with stage IIIA breast cancer treated with surgery alone is dismal, with very few survivors at 10 years. The results are worse for patients with stage IIIB disease treated with surgery alone. The addition of radiation therapy to surgery improves local control but has little impact upon overall survival. The most promising approach thus far is combined modality therapy which utilizes neoadjuvant therapy.

Neoadjuvant therapy or induction therapy was introduced in the early 1970s in an attempt to improve outcome since the results from conventional therapy were not satisfactory. The chemotherapy is delivered prior to local therapy being delivered. The disadvantages are that the patient is not accurately staged, since often the tumor size is reduced and axillary nodal metastases respond to the therapy. In addition, if the disease is not responsive to chemotherapy, local treatment is delayed. The advantages to neoadjuvant chemotherapy are that the chemotherapy is delivered before the vascular supply to the tumor is altered and the patient begins treatment before resistant clones develop. Lastly, the disease can be down-sized, which may then allow for less radical surgery, and patients may become eligible for breast conservation treatment.

When local therapy is delivered initially, the tumor burden is considerably larger when adjuvant chemotherapy is delivered. When neoadjuvant therapy is delivered, the tumor burden is reduced prior to the delivery of locoregional therapy. It is further reduced after the local therapy to allow the adjuvant therapy to act against a much smaller tumor burden.

Studies have evaluated the effects of neoadjuvant chemotherapy on tumor size reduction, axillary lymph node status and the enhanced ability to offer breast conservation therapy. It has been well documented that neoadjuvant chemotherapy results in a reduction in primary tumor size, a reduction in the number of positive axillary lymph nodes and allows women who were not initially candidates for breast conservation to be treated with this type of local/regional treatment.

Significant progress has been made in the treatment of locally advanced breast cancer. However, it is clear that there is room for improvement and the optimal therapy for locally advanced breast cancer has yet to be determined. It is apparent that patients with large breast cancers may become candidates for breast conservation therapy after neoadjuvant therapy without compromising their overall survival; however, this is not standard therapy and should not be offered outside of a clinical trial.

INFLAMMATORY BREAST CANCER

Inflammatory breast cancer was first described in 1814 and the term 'inflammatory breast cancer' was coined in 1924. It falls into the category of stage IIIB breast cancer when there is no evidence of metastatic disease and is considered as locally advanced and inoperable. It accounts for approximately 1–2% of breast cancers at presentation and had been associated with an extremely poor prognosis. According to the SEER data, the incidence of inflammatory breast cancer is higher in African–American women when compared to white and other non-white women. It is characterized by the rapid onset of symptoms with diffuse involvement of the breast. Often, there is no palpable mass and the patient presents with erythema of the breast with skin edema and peau d'orange. Often, the patient experiences a delay in diagnosis due to initial treatment for a mastitis. The diagnosis can be established with either fine needle aspiration cytology, core biopsy or incisional biopsy.

The overall survival for patients treated by local/regional therapy alone has a dismal prognosis, with nearly all patients developing distant metastases. Patients treated by surgery alone have a 5-year survival of <10%. When patients are treated with surgery and radiation therapy, there is improved local control but there is no impact on overall survival.

Due to the poor prognosis and likelihood for distant metastases, patients with inflammatory breast cancer have been treated more successfully with combined modality therapy. A variety of chemotherapy regimens have been employed and the optimal treatment regimen is not known. Patients are generally treated with induction chemotherapy for four cycles or to best response. Local therapy has ranged from surgery alone, surgery plus radiation, radiation plus surgery and radiation alone. After local treatment, patients may then receive maintenance chemotherapy for 1–2 years. Local/regional recurrence rates vary from 8 to 39% and in many instances, follow-up is short. In studies with longer follow-up, disease-free survival ranges from 28 to 59% and overall survival ranges from 30 to 63%. Patients with inflammatory breast cancer may also be candidates for participation in bone marrow transplant/autologous stem cell reinfusion trials. Patients who have had a complete response to chemotherapy have improved disease-free survivals when compared to those who are partial responders.

Bibliography

Cabanes PA, Salmon RJ, Vilcoq JR, *et al.* Value of axillary dissection in addition to lumpectomy and radiotherapy in early breast cancer. *Lancet* 1992;339: 1245–8

Clarke DH, Martinez AA. Identification of patients who are at high risk for locoregional breast cancer recurrence after conservative surgery and radiotherapy: a review article for surgeons, pathologists and radiation and medical oncologists. *J Clin Oncol* 1992; 10:474–83

Fisher B, Redmond C, Poissin R, *et al.* Eight-year results of a randomized clinical trial comparing total mastectomy and lumpectomy with or without irradiation in the treatment of breast cancer. *N Engl J Med* 1989;320:822–8

Frykberg ER, Bland KI. Management of *in situ* and minimally invasive breast carcinoma. *World J Surg* 1994;18:45–57

Haffty BG, Ward B, Pathare P, *et al.* Reappraisal of the role of axillary lymph node dissection in the conservative treatment of breast cancer. *J Clin Oncol* 1997;15:691–700

Jaiyesimi IA, Buzdar AU, Hortobagyi G. Inflammatory breast cancer: a review. *J Clin Oncol* 1992;10: 1014–24

NIH Consensus Conference. Treatment of early-stage breast cancer. *J Am Med Assoc* 1991;265:391–5

Orel SG, Troupin RH, Patterson EA, *et al.* Breast cancer recurrence after lumpectomy and irradiation: role of mammography in detection. *Radiology* 1992;183:201–6

Swallow CJ, Van Zee KJ, Sacchini V, *et al.* Ductal carcinoma *in situ* of the breast: progress and controversy. *Curr Probl Surg* 1996;33:553–608

Radiation treatment for breast cancer: a means of breast conservation

15

S.O. Asbell

Radiation therapy (XRT) should be considered for most patients with carcinoma of the breast if breast conservation is desired. Many states require physicians to offer patients the choice of therapy, i.e. surgery versus radiation therapy, before any treatment is delivered.

Before breast conserving treatment can be offered, the extent or stage of disease must be determined. Criteria for staging appear in *The Manual For Staging of Cancer* and have been accepted by the UICC, Union Against Cancer and the American Joint Committee on Cancer (AJCC) (see Table 15.1). Stages range from limited disease stage 1 through increasing stages with increase in tumor size or lymph node spread up to stage 4, when there is evidence of metastases. Staging utilizes the TNM classification where tumor dimension (T) increases from small size T_1 to T_4 which is associated with fixation, extension through the skin or chest wall, or peau d'orange, i.e. inflammatory carcinoma. The required accountability of lymph node involvement outside the breast extends from no nodal involvement, N_0, N_1 for nodes in the axilla to N_3 for those of the internal mammary chains. Recently, metastasis (M) has included spread to lymph nodes in the supraclavicular fossa, M_1, which is also used to denote other sites of dissemination, for example, to bone, lung and liver. M_0 indicates that there is no metastasis.

Listed in Table 15.1 are several types of breast carcinoma. Ductal carcinoma *in situ* (DCIS), and

Table 15.1 Breast cancer histologic classifications

Ductal
Intraductal (*in situ*) (DCIS)
Invasive with predominant intraductal component
Invasive, NOS (not otherwise specified)
Comedo
Inflammatory
Medullary with lymphocytic infiltrate*
Mucinous (colloid)*
Papillary*
Scirrhous
Tubular*
Other

Lobular
In situ (LCIS)
Invasive with predominant *in situ* component
Invasive (2)

Nipple
Paget's disease NOS
Paget's disease with intraductal carcinoma
Paget's disease with invasive ductal carcinoma

Undifferentiated carcinoma

*Favorable histologic type

infiltrating ductal and lobular types may be treated with radiation therapy. Rarely the breast may be involved with other tumors such as melanoma, lymphoma or sarcoma. The latter three types of tumor require different combinations of chemotherapy and different doses of radiotherapy and will not be covered in this chapter.

WHO ARE CANDIDATES FOR BREAST CONSERVING RADIATION TREATMENT?

Patients with DCIS or invasive carcinoma of the breast stage I or II (those with minimal primary tumors and those with limited numbers of axillary nodes) are good candidates for breast salvage with radiation treatment after lumpectomy. If surgery is refused, radiation may be used alone to achieve a reasonable chance of local control. However, higher doses are required with less chance of local control and good cosmesis. Patients with stage III and IV breast cancers may, under certain circumstances, receive whole breast irradiation followed by mastectomy or chest wall irradiation after mastectomy. Some cases have such advanced local disease that complete surgical excision cannot be performed and radiation with chemo/hormonal therapy is the sole treatment.

Knowledge of age, stage, menopausal status, hormonal receptor status and other pathologic factors need to be assessed in order to decide if chemotherapy and/or hormonal therapy should be given in conjunction with radiotherapy. Usually, women with three or more involved axillary lymph nodes are treated before, during and frequently after XRT with multi-agent chemotherapy. Several regimens are available with the optimal chemotherapy being controversial. However, a combination of cytoxan, methotrexate and 5-fluorouracil, the so-called CMF regimen, has become very common. Other regimens that are used will be discussed in the chapter on adjuvant therapy. The timing of chemotherapy is controversial with data supporting its use either prior to radiation or after.

As for hormonal treatment, currently, tamoxifen, an anti-estrogen, is usually offered as the first hormonal manipulation. Because of an increased risk of endometrial carcinoma, it is currently recommended that its use be continued for at least 2 years but no more than 5. As yet, studies regarding its efficacy and risks have not been finalized. Most agree that postmenopausal women with estrogen and progesterone receptor (ER/PR) positive tumors >1 cm and/or three or more involved axillary lymph nodes should take tamoxifen. Tamoxifen is frequently used along with chemotherapy if the lymph nodes are involved. There are several other effective hormonal agents or manipulations such as oophorectomy, which may be offered in premenopausal women. The details of the use of hormones and chemotherapy will be discussed in Chapter 16.

Patients with advanced cancer, stages 3 and 4 that have large tumors, >5 cm T_3 lesions or tumors with direct extension to the skin and chest wall (T_4) should be considered for XRT combined with mastectomy, chemotherapy and/or hormonal management. For these patients, conservation of the breast is a far less important feature than the attempt at long-term tumor control.

Before the patient can choose breast-conserving therapy, she must be made aware of the indications, contraindications, the relative contraindications, risks and benefits of this treatment option. Patients who received prior radiation for other malignancies in the region of the breast usually should not be considered for irradiation. Pregnant women should not be irradiated but breast-conserving surgery may be scheduled during the third trimester of pregnancy with the radiation administered after the delivery. Breast-conserving therapy is not always well tolerated by the elderly and should be considered on an individual basis. It can be considered a relative contraindication. Active collagen-vascular diseases may also be considered a relative contraindication as XRT may not be well tolerated, and therefore management should be individualized.

Before undergoing a course of radiotherapy, patients must be aware of the cosmetic results anticipated. Those with large breasts may note decreasing breast size after several years and must anticipate asymmetry (see Figure 15.1). On the other hand, patients with smaller-sized breasts may show little change after treatment with excellent cosmesis (see Figure 15.2), as long as the surgery left the breast without significant

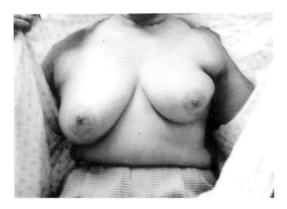

Figure 15.1 Asymmetry due to shrinkage 2 years after the breast was irradiated

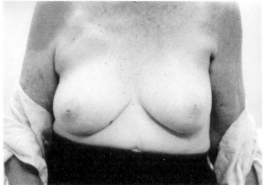

Figure 15.2 The irradiated breast is indistinguishable from normal 2 years after treatment

loss of volume or contour. Women with very small breasts must consider that they may be left with little breast tissue after lumpectomy when contemplating breast-conserving management, as the cosmetic difference from mastectomy may be small. If a quadrantectomy has to be performed to remove tumor, by virtue of large tumor or small breast size, cosmesis is usually not fully satisfactory. A mastectomy may also then be recommended. Patients with multifocal disease (two or more tumors in different quadrants) should have a mastectomy. Although radiation therapy has been found useful for localized DCIS, there have been a few studies initiated recently to test the role of radiation therapy in the face of diffuse intraductal malignancy.

After tumor removal, a mammogram should be obtained before radiation is initiated to prove there is no residual disease and to provide a baseline. Thus, the radiologist can be assured future changes on mammography have developed subsequent to lumpectomy and radiation treatment.

Before radiation therapy is started, the patient should be immobilized in such a way to be able to repeat the exact position daily without major discomfort as the position must be held for about 5 min daily. The treatment conditions including the immobilized patient must be simulated so that treatment planning decisions may be made by the therapeutic radiologist

regarding the need for use of tissue compensation. Treatments should be 5 days a week.

The terms for describing radiation dose has changed in the past few years. Radiation doses are frequently described in Gray (Gy) rather than rads, where 1 centigray (cGy) is equal to 1 rad or 102 joules of energy/kg, i.e. absorbed dose per unit mass. The dose of radiation is usually between 180 and 200 cGy per fraction each day until the minimal total dose of 4500–5000 cGy has been delivered. In the USA, patients treated at centers which have received accreditation from the American College of Radiology or the American College of Radiation Oncology may be more assured that the treatment techniques have been surveyed and are well within the acceptable standards of care.

Radiation is usually given to the entire intact breast after lumpectomy as prophylaxis for any subclinical disease outside the lumpectomy site. Curative radiation therapy usually consists of treatment directed medially and laterally to the breast with supervoltage beams of photon energy of 4–6 Mev. The angled breast fields are called tangents as they skim the chest wall and ribcage without large volumes of lung being included (see Figure 15.3a, b). Using these techniques, long-term survival is expected. For early tumors with no lymph node involvement, a 10-year survival of 83–91% and a disease-free survival of 79–88% are expected. For those with lymph node involvement, 10-year disease-free

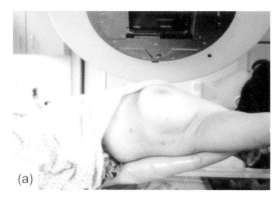

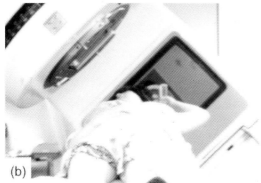

Figure 15.3 Patient in position for radiation treatment to medial and lateral tangential breast fields

survival is 71% and at 20 years only 66%. With two to four lymph nodes involved, the survival rates drop to 62 and 56%, respectively, and with more than four lymph nodes, 47 and 43%. Radiation results after lumpectomy have been found equal to those of mastectomy in patients whose disease has been limited to the breast or into the adjacent lymphatics with less than three axillary lymph nodes involved. When more than three axillary lymph nodes are involved, patients should receive not only radiation to the breast but also to the supraclavicular fossa and apex of the axilla. The supraclavicular fossa is usually treated from an anterior direction only and abutted to the tangential breast fields such that there is no overlap of treatment fields. Even patients who have distant metastatic disease are treated with breast radiation to control the disease locally, with minimal doses usually in the range of 4500–5000 cGy. However, higher doses are frequently required.

A dose of 5000 cGy to the tumor bed is not felt to be curative by many radiation oncologists. There is controversy about the need for boosting the lumpectomy site, i.e. tumor bed, with additional radiation. Frequently, recurrences are at the area of initial biopsy, so boosting this zone might diminish the risk. The boost may be given in the form of daily electron beam therapy or less commonly with a radioactive implant (brachytherapy). If brachytherapy is used, it may be prior to or at the conclusion of the external beam radiation therapy. Afterloading radioactive implants, frequently iridium-192 (^{192}Ir), limit the radiation exposure to within a few centimeters of their placement in the patient. Usually doses are in the range of 1000–1600 cGy. Standards have not been established. Electrons up to 15 Mev, depending on the depth needed, may be used in contrast to photons of 4–6 Mev, thus sparing deep radiation to the breast or lung. The depth of interest required may be determined if clips have been placed at surgery or by using the hematoma site found on ultrasound. If electron beam therapy is chosen at the conclusion of the radiation to the entire breast, there is an additional week to 10 days of therapy. Usually, a daily dose of 180–200 cGy is used for an additional 1000–2000 cGy, bringing the total dose to the tumor bed to 6000–6600 cGy.

If treatment is planned to areas around the breast, i.e. the supraclavicular fossa, a dose similar to the breast, between 4500 and 5000 cGy, through a single anterior field with matched lines and angles to the breast tangential fields is used.

More advanced tumors that have skin involvement must have special calculations performed to ensure that an adequate skin dose has been administered. Tissue-equivalent material called bolus consisting of rice bags, stacks of gauze, or superflab is placed over the breast to increase radiation to the skin below.

When a patient has more advanced disease and no surgery is planned, treatment usually includes the entire breast, the supraclavicular fossa, and the axilla.

IMMEDIATE EFFECTS OF XRT ON SKIN AND MANAGEMENT

Care of the breast during and after treatment is customarily managed by the radiation oncologist. Usually, at the completion of radiation therapy, the skin has become dry, scaly and hyperpigmented. The dry desquamation is similar to that of skin peeling from sunburn. Occasionally, a moist desquamation may develop near the completion of treatment which takes 7–10 days to heal. It is especially prone to occur in areas of friction such as the axilla and inframammary fold, especially when patients have large breasts. Furthermore, the nipple may become sensitive after radiation. Treatment with topical steroids frequently decreases the patient's discomfort. Also, Vaseline gauze may assist the patient in getting through the remainder of therapy should a moist reaction develop before treatment completion. The primary physician should not allow the course of therapy to be interrupted, as cure could be compromised. Once the course has been completed, usually silvadene, which contains silver, may be used without fear of interference with the proper radiation reaction. It frequently assists in healing, most of which occurs in the first 7–10 days. The cosmetic appearance of the breast becomes similar to the untreated breast once desquamation has stopped and sufficient time has passed, usually a few months. Tattoos are frequently placed at the center and margins of the radiation fields. This may be useful if field reconstruction is necessary and should future planning be warranted.

POST-MASTECTOMY RADIOTHERAPY INDICATIONS

Radiation therapy may also be used postoperatively. The chest wall and supraclavicular fossa are usually treated after mastectomy when there is a high probability of chest wall tumor

recurrence or supraclavicular adenopathy. Indications for chest wall radiation include:

1. Large primary, i.e. greater than 5 cm.

2. Skin or chest wall involvement with tumor.

3. More than three axillary lymph nodes involved with tumor.

4. Incomplete tumor removal or positive margins.

5. Recurrence on the chest wall in skin or subcutaneous tissue.

Indications for supraclavicular fossa treatment include:

1. Supraclavicular adenopathy.

2. Multiple axillary nodes or tumor outside of the nodes and adjacent tissues.

3. Tumor extension into the supraclavicular fossa.

Radiation may be given safely after breast reconstruction with silicone or saline implants. Cosmesis may be affected and capsular fibrosis with associated pain may occasionally necessitate implant removal.

RADIATION THERAPY FOR RECURRENCE

Radiotherapy may be used to gain permanent control of chest wall recurrences either after excision or biopsy. The dose required is similar to that of primary breast radiotherapy. However, if the tumor is bulky, it may require additional doses of 1000–2000 cGy. Thus, doses may range from 4500 to 7000 cGy and occasionally 8000 cGy to smaller areas. Treatment is protracted over several weeks, usually at a dose rate of 180–200 cGy per day. Some places use larger daily doses to accomplish the goal faster, but at greater risk for side-effects and more acute reaction to the therapy. In some institutions, treatment is hyperfractionated with two or more treatments given daily so that the total daily dose exceeds the usual. The patient may better tolerate this course, especially if higher doses are required to clear disease from a substantial area. Usually, photons of 4–6 Mev are used; however, electrons of varying energies may be appropriately utilized for part or for the entire course of therapy. Treating prophylactically usually results in better control than when there is bulky tumor present, which requires higher doses. Some places take advantage of radiotherapy along with hyperthermia, when doses usually vary from the standard as well as the fractionation schedule. Frequently, hormonal and/or chemotherapy is administered simultaneously.

COMPLICATIONS OF XRT TO THE BREAST AND CHEST WALL

When local radiation is applied to the breast, supraclavicular fossa, and/or axilla, patients do not usually experience nausea, hair loss, nor diminution of their blood count. The skin reaction secondary to radiation has been described earlier in this chapter. When doses in excess of 6000 cGy are used, local ulceration may occur and take a long time to heal. Late fat necrosis may occur many months after radiation is completed and confuse the observer with tumor recurrence. The latter is very uncommon and must be considered a late complication. Arm edema may occur in as high as 12% of patients usually after axillary dissection and radiation therapy. Other relatively rare (3%) late complications which occur from months to years after radiation include: fractured ribs in the region of the field of radiation (portal), pericarditis if the heart is included in the portal, and pneumonitis from including a portion of the lung. Brachial plexopathy may occur if high dose radiation is given to the supraclavicular fossa. Complications may be augmented when radiation is given simultaneously or in tandem with chemotherapy. This is especially true with drugs which are radiosensitizers or enhancers of radiation effects such as adriamycin and methotrexate. The effects of Taxol, and its relatives, have not yet been fully studied.

Bibliography

Devita VT, Hellman S, Rosenberg SA. *Cancer Principles and Practice of Oncology*, 4th Edition. Philadelphia: J.B. Lippincott Co., 1993

Harris JR, Lippman ME, Morrow M, *et al*. *Diseases of the Breast*. Philadelphia: J.B. Lippincott Co., 1996

Kuske RR, Schuster R, Klein E, *et al*. Radiotherapy and breast reconstruction: clinical results and dosimetry. *Int J Radiat Oncol Biol Physiol* 1991;21:339–46

Moore PM, Kinne DW. The surgical management of primary invasive breast cancer. *CA A Cancer Journal for Clinicians* 1995;45:279–88

Perez CA, Brady LW. *Principles and Practice of Radiation Oncology*, 2nd Edition. Philadelphia: J.B. Lippincott Co., 1992

Adjuvant therapy

16

S.O. Asbell

DEFINITION OF ADJUVANT THERAPY

Adjuvant breast cancer therapy is chemotherapy and/or radiotherapy and/or hormonal therapy given in addition to tumor removal, to decrease the chance of recurrence or distant spread. It may be used before, during or after radiation and similarly before or after mastectomy under certain circumstances.

BACKGROUND OF ADJUVANT RADIATION THERAPY

Radiation therapy has been used as definitive therapy, as well as adjuvant therapy after lumpectomy. Randomized trials have shown its value in diminishing recurrence.

Once a tumor has been debulked via lumpectomy, there is still a risk of local recurrence at the site of lumpectomy and within the breast which is significantly reduced by 5000–6000 cGy of photon radiation. Even after mastectomy, a similar dose is frequently used to diminish the risk of recurrence when there is a risk of microscopic disease which may remain after removal of large tumors or one with local aggressive features.

BACKGROUND AND TYPES OF HORMONAL THERAPY AND/OR CHEMOTHERAPY

Our understanding of the mechanisms of action of hormonal agents in normal and pathologic breast tissue has expanded dramatically over the last 30 years. The identification of specific receptors for estrogens, progestins, androgens, and glucocorticoids led to the elucidation of the cascade of events that results in the intended effect of steroid hormones. The ability to identify and quantitate estrogen and progesterone receptor expression in individual tissues was soon followed by clinical correlations that established the diagnostic and predictive importance of these elements in the management of metastatic and primary breast carcinoma.

The background thinking about adjuvant chemotherapy or hormonal therapy for the management of invasive breast cancer is based on the investigations of many physicians who noted that only a minority of patients were cured after radical surgery or radical radiotherapy. These were in patients who did not harbor sub-clinical metastases. Those who failed to respond succumbed to widespread metastases. Thus, the plan of using combined modality (i.e. radiation, surgery and chemotherapy) therapy to control both regional and systemic disease was born.

The initial trials of adjuvant systemic hormonal therapy involved surgical oophorectomy or radiation castration. Later, single agent chemotherapy was tried. These early clinical trials were with inadequate numbers and questionable statistical usefulness, but it became clear that ovarian function ablation prolonged disease-free and sometimes overall survival in premenopausal women. By the early 1970s, more sound scientific principles of chemotherapy became available and prospective randomized clinical trials began. The completion of several randomized clinical trials that compared tamoxifen with estrogens, aminoglutethimide, progestins, and oophorectomy soon established

Table 16.1 Prognostic factors in patients with lymph node-negative breast cancer and probability of recurrence at 5 years

Prognostic factors	5 year recurrence (%)
Aneuploid, high cathepsin D	>50
High HER-2, estrogen-receptor positive, <3 cm in size	>50
Estrogen-receptor negative	>30
High S-phase fraction	30
Nuclear grade 3 (poor)	≥25
Estrogen-receptor positive	≥25
Nuclear grade 2 (intermediate)	≥25
Aneuploid	≥25
Diploid	<15
Tumor size <2 cm	<15
Low S-phase fraction	<15
Nuclear grade 1 (good)	<15
Tumor size <1 cm	<15
Non-invasive	≥1

the prominent role of this agent as the treatment of choice for hormone-responsive metastatic breast carcinoma. Today, anti-estrogens in general, and tamoxifen in particular, are considered the first-line treatment of choice for hormone-responsive metastatic breast carcinoma, and hormonal receptor-positive primary breast carcinoma that requires adjuvant systemic treatment. The discovery of estrogen (ER) and progesterone (PR) receptors in cancer tissue helped define who would best be served with hormonal therapy, ER positive disease being an indicator for use of hormonal manipulation. Both adjuvant chemotherapy and tamoxifen were found to improve disease-free and overall survival rates in certain populations of breast cancer patients.

In the USA, early national invasive breast cancer clinical studies were based on stage. Those which involved axillary lymph nodes represented less favorable status, higher stage and they benefited from the use of chemotherapy with a reduction of recurrence and death from disease. It was also found that many patients benefited from tamoxifen. Which patients could profit from hormonal manipulation with tamoxifen and perhaps chemotherapy as well?

The National Surgical Adjuvant Breast and Bowel Project (NSABP) studied the use of tamoxifen. They established that in women with ER/PR-positive status tamoxifen was beneficial. There was delay in initiating chemotherapy studies for those in whom this favorable prognosis existed after surgery, especially those with negative nodes. Was the possible development of late hematologic malignancy that could result from alkylating agents worth the risk? It was not until the early 1980s that they finally decided that even node-negative women might profit from adjuvant chemotherapy. In the more recently published results of the NSABP B-20 study, they evaluated women with more favorable disease, i.e. axillary lymph node-negative and ER-positive disease. Women were eligible if they had mastectomy or lumpectomy followed by 5000 cGy of external beam radiotherapy (XRT) directed to the breast. They found a greater reduction of ipsilateral local and regional breast recurrence as well as a reduction of distant sites of spread when tamoxifen was used with combination chemotherapy with either cyclophosphamide, methotrexate and 5 fluorouracil (CMF), or methotrexate and 5 fluorouracil (MF) than for those randomized to tamoxifen alone.

Currently, at least three national studies are open assessing tamoxifen as an adjuvant treatment in invasive breast cancer patients. One is B-29 where tamoxifen is used alone or in combination with either octreotide or adriamycin cyclophosphamide (AC). These patients have negative axillary nodes estrogen receptor-positive disease. Also, there is B-21 for occult breast cancer with node-negative disease treated by lumpectomy followed by a randomization between tamoxifen alone or in combination with XRT, or XRT alone. Because it has been discovered that tamoxifen may have activity in estrogen receptor-negative patients, the NSABP has opened another trial with tamoxifen for estrogen receptor and node-negative women with breast cancer. This trial, B-23, in addition to lumpectomy, randomizes between CMF with

Table 16.2 Summary for standard adjuvant systemic therapy (non-protocol)

Patient status		Adjuvant therapy	
Age in years	Estrogen-receptor status	Hormone or tamoxifen therapy	Chemotherapy
Premenopause			
<50	Negative	No	Yes
<50	Positive	Yes	Yes
<50	Unknown	No	Yes
Postmenopause			
≥50	Negative	No	Yes
≥50	Positive	Yes	Yes/No
≥50	Unknown	Yes	Yes

and without tamoxifen, and AC with and without tamoxifen.

The Early Breast Cancer Trial Collaborative Group published a meta-analysis and demonstrated that multi-agent chemotherapy was more effective than single agent in reducing death and recurrence. Attempts were then made to find the best combinations to use in the adjuvant setting, based on all prognostic factors known at the time. Under the leadership of Bernard Fisher, the NSABP studied various combinations of chemotherapy and tamoxifen. Early studies showed the benefit of CMF. Also, MF was an effective combination in the NSABP B-13 study. However, those patients with very aggressive disease, those with estrogen receptor-negative disease, or multiple axillary lymph nodes seemed to show less response to these regimens, but more to the more potentially toxic combinations first found effective in metastatic disease. Combinations with cyclophosphamide and either anthracyclines, for example adriamycin, doxorubicin or epirubicin, have been used. One of the most popular combinations found to decrease relapse-free survival was high dose chemotherapy with cyclophosphamide, Adriamycin® (Pharmacia & Upjohn, Kalamazoo, MI, USA) and 5 fluorouracil (FAC). The risk of cardiac toxicity from adriamycin is reduced to <1% if the total cumulative dose is less than 400 mg/m^2. However, newer less toxic agents of similar biologic

activity have been developed and are in current trials. Dexrazoxane® (Pharmacia & Upjohn, Kalamazoo, MI, USA) is currently in trial to allow more toxic doses of chemotherapy without the fear of cardiac damage. Also, other new medications such as Taxol® (Bristol-Myers Squibb, Princeton, NJ, USA) are in trials to discern if they are more efficacious in the adjuvant setting. The NSABP is currently conducting an aggressive study for patients with T1-3, N1, M0 disease, which is B-28, a Randomized Trial Evaluating the Worth of Taxol Following Adriamycin/Cyclophosphamide in Breast Cancer Patients with Positive Axillary Nodes. As other agents are found to be effective in metastatic disease (see Chapter 17), they too may be tried.

Very aggressive adjuvant therapy has been designed for breast cancer patients with >10 nodes in the axilla because they carry such a poor prognosis. The Eastern Cooperative Oncology Group (ECOG) developed a Phase III study of adjuvant chemotherapy versus high dose chemotherapy and autologous bone marrow/stem cell transplantation in stages II and III breast cancer. Granulocyte stimulatory factor (GCSF), is now available and is used to help stimulate regrowth of bone marrow when toxicity from chemotherapy has suppressed it. There are several other factors for red blood cells and platelets available.

The conclusions of NSABP B-13 and B-19 confirmed that premenopausal and

Table 16.3 Suggested adjuvant systemic therapy for node-negative breast cancer patients outside clinical trials

Breast cancer patient with	Adjuvant therapy
Favorable histology* ≥2 cm	Yes
Invasive ductal/lobular ≥1 cm	Yes
Favorable histology <2 cm (tubular, mucinous)	No
Invasive cancer <1 cm	No
Microinvasive disease	No
Non-invasive (DCIS, LCIS)	No

*See Table 15.1 for favorable histology

postmenopausal, both ER(+) and (–), profited from chemotherapeutic regimens but for CMF there was a slight advantage in those <49 years old. For stage II breast cancer the PR(+) may have greater prognostic significance than the ER status suggests.

The search for refinement in therapy and for whom hormonal therapy, chemotherapy or their combination should be used, led us to the use of prognostic indicators. In addition to those listed in Table 16.1, thymidine-labeling index, tumor micro vessel density, C-erb, B-2, C-myc, p53 expression and peritumoral lymphatic vessel invasion may also be prognostic indicators.

From the list in Table 16.3, patients can be divided into groups with high and low risk of developing recurrence or metastasis and their therapy chosen accordingly. This is a simplified list for understanding risk but one factor should not be used alone. The low risk group has <15% 5-year chance of recurrence. Favorable histologies are listed in Table 15.1.

Which patients are not routinely offered adjuvant chemotherapy or hormonal therapy?

As of 1998, patients not offered routine chemotherapy or hormonal therapy are those with stage I tumors <1 cm and favorable histology, i.e. with medullary, mucinous, papillary tubular carcinoma. There is no defined role for adjuvant chemo- or hormonal therapy for ductal

carcinoma *in situ* (DCIS); however, NSABP B-24 trials which have been completed, but not yet analyzed, compared the treatment of women with positive microscopic margins after local excision for DCIS with postoperative XRT and tamoxifen versus placebo for lobular carcinoma *in situ*.

For lobular carcinoma *in situ* (LCIS), which is associated with a high risk of developing invasive cancer, there is no established adjuvant therapy. The NSABP had a trial of tamoxifen for the prevention of invasive cancer which closed in September 1997. Results are not yet available.

TIMING OF ADJUVANT THERAPY

It appears that the timing of adjuvant therapy could be important in obtaining optimal results in terms of relapse-free and overall survival, with its initiation early in the course of management being more favorable. Contrasting data from retrospective analysis support radiation both before and after chemotherapy. With these conflicting results, it is difficult to determine which is more efficacious, but more recent data have convinced many medical oncologists of the need to initiate chemotherapy usually before radiation. There is one report which suggests that even starting tamoxifen 2 years after the diagnosis may result in some therapeutic benefit by prolonging disease-free survival. The appropriate time for the initiation of tamoxifen before or after radiation therapy for lumpectomy patients remains undefined.

DURATION OF HORMONAL THERAPY AND/OR CHEMOTHERAPY

How long should adjuvant hormonal or chemotherapy be maintained? Initially most studies required 1–2 years because of cumulative side-effects and non-compliance. National studies have been performed to help substantiate exactly how long therapy should be administered. In early studies, multi-agent chemotherapy if administered for less than 6 months produced inferior disease-free and overall survival. Later, with more aggressive agents, four cycles of AC were found to be equivalent to six cycles of CMF in one study. The duration of therapy will depend on the agents used and newer combinations will obviously vary.

As for the duration of hormonal therapy, three clinical experiments have demonstrated that tamoxifen has a long-term suppressive effect on proliferation of breast cancer and if the medication is stopped, tumor regrowth occurs. On this basis, the use of tamoxifen had been increased in adjuvant hormonal therapy protocols.

The Early Breast Cancer Trialists' Collaborative Group analyzed the results of 55 randomized trials comparing treatment with, and without, adjuvant tamoxifen before 1990; 37 000 women were included, 8000 of whom had ER-negative status. Among these, the overall effects of tamoxifen appeared to be small. They are not included in the following statistical analysis of recurrence and total mortality which was restricted to the remaining women (18 000 with ER-positive tumors, plus nearly 12 000 more with untested tumors, of which an estimated 8000 would have been ER-positive). For trials of 1 year, 2 years, and 5 years duration of adjuvant tamoxifen, the proportional recurrence reductions produced among these 30 000 women, during about 10 years of follow-up, were 21% (SD = 3), 29% (SD = 2) and 47% (SD = 3), respectively, with a highly significant trend towards greater effect with longer treatment $(\chi^2_1 = 52.0, 2p = 0.00001)$. The corresponding proportional mortality reductions were 12% (SD = 3), 17% (SD = 3) and 26% (SD = 4), respectively, and again the test for trends was significant $(\chi^2_1 = 8.8, 2p = 0.003)$. The absolute improvement in recurrence was greater during the first 5 years, whereas the improvement in survival grew steadily larger throughout the first 10 years. The proportional mortality reactions were similar for women with node-positive and node-negative disease, but the absolute mortality reductions were greater in node-positive women. In the trials of approximately 5 years of adjuvant tamoxifen the absolute improvements in the 10-year survival were 10.9% (SD = 2.5) for node-positive (61.4% vs. 50.5% survival, $2p < 0.00001$) and 5.6% (SD = 1.3) for node-negative (78.9% vs. 73.3% survival, $2p = 0.00001$). These benefits appeared to be largely irrespective of age, menopausal status, daily tamoxifen dose (which was generally 20 mg), and of whether chemotherapy had been given to both groups.

Results from the National Surgical Adjuvant Breast and Bowel Project (NSABP) protocol B-14, evaluated 5 versus 10 years of tamoxifen as adjuvant therapy for early stage breast cancer and found no advantage to continue >5 years in node-negative ER positive cancer. The risks of therapy are listed in the section on toxicity.

HOW TO DETERMINE APPROPRIATE THERAPY

It has been generally accepted that all patients with node-positive primary breast cancer or stage III disease, except those with significant coexistent morbidity should receive adjuvant systemic treatment. Women with ER(+) disease, unless the tumor is <1 cm, usually receive tamoxifen in their course of treatment for up to 5 years. Furthermore, many patients with node-positive breast cancer who have adverse prognostic indicators (see Table 16.1) which place them in the moderate to high-risk category should also receive adjuvant systemic therapy. Many trials are open to define the best therapy for women with breast cancer. Patients should be encouraged to participate to help define the least toxic best chance for disease control.

TOXICITIES OF HORMONAL THERAPY AND/OR CHEMOTHERAPY

The toxicities of hormone therapy and chemotherapy are discussed in detail in Chapter 17.

Bibliography

The American Cancer Society 1996 Advisory Committee on Diet, Nutrition, and Cancer Prevention. American Cancer Society guidelines on diet, nutrition, and cancer prevention: reducing the risk of cancer with healthy food choices and physical activity. *CA A Cancer Journal for Clinicians* 1996;46:325–42

Cancer Fax (National Cancer Institute Cancer Data Base) Information from PDQ for Health Professionals. Breast Cancer. *PDQ,* 208/00013, 57/98

Devita VT, Hellman S, Rosenberg SA. *Cancer Principles and Practice of Oncology,* 5th Edition. Philadelphia: J.B. Lippincott Co., 1996

Early Breast Cancer Trialists' Collaborative Group. Part I: Systemic treatment of early breast cancer by hormonal, cytotoxic, or immune therapy: 133 randomized trials involving 31,000 recurrences and 24,000 deaths among 75,000 women. *Lancet* 1992; 339:1–15

Early Breast Cancer Trialists' Collaborative Group. Part II: Systemic treatment of early breast cancer by hormonal, cytotoxic, or immune therapy: 133 randomized trials involving 31,000 recurrences and 24,000 deaths among 75,000 women. *Lancet* 1992; 339:71–85

Early Breast Cancer Trialists' Collaborative Group. Tamoxifen for early breast cancer: an overview of the randomized trials. *Lancet* 1998;351:1451–67

Fisher B, Dignam J, Mamounas EP, *et al.* Sequential methotrexate and fluorouracil for the treatment of node-negative breast cancer patients with estrogen receptor-negative tumors: eight-year results from National Surgical Adjuvant Breast and Bowel Project (NSABP) B-13 and first report of findings from NSABP B-19 comparing methotrexate and fluorouracil with conventional cyclophosphamide, methotrexate and fluorouracil (see comments) *J Clin Oncol* 1996;14:1971–3

Fisher B, Dignam J, Wolmark N, *et al.* Tamoxifen and chemotherapy for lymph-node negative, estrogen receptor-positive breast cancer (see comments). *J Natl Cancer Inst* 1997;89:1652–4

Harris JR, Lippman ME, Morrow M, *et al. Diseases of the Breast.* Philadelphia: J.B. Lippincott Co., 1996

Hortobagyi GN. Progress in endocrine therapy for breast carcinoma. *Cancer* 1998;83:1–6

Metastatic breast cancer/palliation   17

S.O. Asbell

HORMONES, CHEMOTHERAPY, ANTIBODY TREATMENT, RADIATION THERAPY AND SURGERY

Once the breast cancer has disseminated outside the origin of the breast, chest wall, and adjacent lymph nodes, cure is unlikely and systemic treatment must be considered. Usually, the management chosen depends on:

1. The age of the patient.

2. The ER/PR status.

3. The location of the metastasis.

4. The patient's willingness to accept the side-effects and toxicity of the treatment option.

5. The quality of life the patient is willing to accept or that could be anticipated.

6. The quantity of life anticipated.

The therapy chosen may be hormonal, chemotherapeutic, radiation, or some combination. There are also some interventional and/or surgical procedures which at times must be considered.

Lung, liver, and other visceral metastases are usually treated with chemotherapy, occasionally with hormonal manipulation. Bone marrow or stem cell transplants may be considered for highly selective patients. Palliative radiotherapy should be considered when local treatment could relieve symptoms. When lymph nodal groups, either close to the original lesion or at metastatic sites, such as porta hepatis or mediastinum, cause obstruction, systemic treatment as well as local radiation, either simultaneously or in tandem, should be considered. If the patient is ER/PR positive and is experiencing painful bony metastasis, hormonal therapy may be the initial therapy tried.

HORMONAL THERAPY

Hormonal therapies utilized alone or in combination with chemotherapy and/or radiation therapy include:

1. Prednisone or dexamethasone.

2. Aminoglutethimide.

3. Estradiol or conjugated or esterified estrogens.

4. Medroxyprogesterone or megestrol (anti-estrogen).

5. Methyltestosterone or testolactone or testosterone.

6. Tamoxifen (anti-estrogen) (Novaldex®, Zeneca Inc, Wilmington, DE, USA).

7. Toremifene (anti-estrogen) (Fareston®, Orion Corp., Espoo, Finland).

8. Anastrozole (anti-estrogen/aromatase inhibitor) (Arimidex®, Zeneca Inc, Wilmington, DE, USA).

9. Letrozole (anti-estrogen/aromatase inhibitor) (Femara®, Novartis Pharmaceuticals Corp., East Hanover, NJ, USA).

Recently, Fareston (toremifene), a new anti-estrogen, has become available and behaves similarly to tamoxifen. Arimidex and Femara are also newly available in the USA market. If the patient responded to the first hormonal treatment, then as the disease becomes resistant, another form of hormonal manipulation may be tried with success. For example, after use of tamoxifen, Megace® (Bristol-Myers Squibb, Princeton, NJ, USA) may be successful for some time. The newer agents, Arimidex or Femara, (aromatase inhibitors) are felt to be more effective than Megace for their anti-estrogen behavior. Also included in hormonal manipulation is treatment with aminoglutethimide and hydrocortisone. Although ovarian ablation is still employed in some centers for reasons of cost and expediency, hormonal approaches with better therapeutic ratios are preferred. Synthetic androgens (fluoxymesterone) are used in patients with persistently hormone-responsive tumors as fourth-line therapy, after anti-estrogens, aromatase inhibitors, and progestins.

Side-effects and toxicity of hormonal therapy

Each hormonal agent has specific side-effects. For example, progestational agents have minimal side-effects but may cause fluid retention and pain flare in-patients with metastasis. Estrogens have limited use because of the risk of uterine and vaginal adenocarcinoma. Their side-effects include change in libido, fluid retention, edema, and a slight risk of thrombophlebitis and hypercalcemia.

Tamoxifen has similar side-effects to estrogen; these include hot flashes, menstrual dysfunction (abnormal uterine or extramenstrual bleeding), vaginal discharge, nausea, vomiting, hypercalcemia, fluid retention and weight gain. Clonidine may ameliorate the hot flashes in some patients. Megace has also been used successfully. Some patients have depressive moods. Early menopause caused by adjuvant therapy can increase the early onset of osteoporosis and adverse changes in the serum lipoprotein profile. While some patients may exhibit thrombocytopenia or decrease in antithrombin III or fibrinogen, others have shown an increase of thrombosis and other cardiovascular events. Benign ovarian cyst development may be associated with tamoxifen. There have been recent reports of an increased risk of endometrial carcinoma in women taking tamoxifen. The incidence of endometrial cancer was approximately doubled in trials of 1 or 2 years of tamoxifen and approximately quadrupled in trials of 5 years of tamoxifen (although the number of cases was small and these ratios were not significantly different from each other). However, the absolute decrease in contralateral breast cancer was about twice as large as the absolute increase in the incidence of endometrial cancer. Thus, the risk seems outweighed by the potential gain. Most patients are advised to remain on tamoxifen for 5 years as per NSABP B-14. There have been a few rare cases of retinopathy. Also, secondary tumors derived from the liver and ovaries have been rarely reported. Most patients, however, have few side-effects.

With androgens, virilization, hirsutism, acne, clitoral hypertrophy, and amenorrhea may occur. Aminoglutethimide and the aromatase inhibitors have acute side-effects which include rash, lethargy, orthostatic hypotension, and hypothyroidism.

CHEMOTHERAPEUTIC THERAPIES

If treatment with hormonal manipulation is not anticipated to have a high probability of success for ER/PR-negative patients, usually multiple-agent chemotherapy is tried. There is a large list of effective chemotherapeutic agents and combinations to consider. The use of these agents is not exclusively for ER/PR-negative patients. Some of the currently used chemotherapeutic agents are:

1. Carboplatin (Paraplatin®, Bristol-Myers Squibb, Princeton, NJ, USA) and cisplatin (Platinol®, Bristol-Myers Squibb, NJ, USA).

2. Cyclophosphamide (Cytoxan®, Bristol-Myers Squibb, NJ, USA).

3. Docetaxel (Taxotere®, Rhône-Poulenc Rorer Pharmaceuticals, Collegeville, PA, USA).

4. Doxorubicin (Adriamycin®, Pharmacia & Upjohn, Kalamazoo, MI, USA).

5. Epirubicin (not available in the USA).

6. 5-Fluorouracil.

7. Gemcitabine (Gemzar®, Eli Lilly & Co., Indianapolis, IN, USA).

8. Melphalan (Alkeran®, Glaxo Wellcome, NC, USA).

9. Methotrexate.

10. Mitomycin (Mutamycin®, Bristol-Myers Squibb, NJ, USA).

11. Mitoxantrone (Novantrone®, Immunex Corp., Seattle, WA, USA).

12. Paclitaxel (Taxol).

13. Vincristine (Oncovin®, Eli Lilly & Co., IN, USA).

14. Vinorelbine Tartrate (Navelbine®, Glaxo Wellcome, NC, USA).

Combinations of therapeutic agents are frequently abbreviated. Some of the most commonly used acronyms are presented in Chapter 16.

Side-effects and toxicity of chemotherapy

Side-effects and toxicity of many chemotherapy agents include nausea, vomiting, anorexia, alopecia, mucositis, leukopenia, neutropenia, thrombocytopenia, infection and amenorrhea. Alopecia occurs in approximately 50% of the patients when combination chemotherapy (cyclophosphamide, methotrexate and 5-fluorouracil; CMF) is given. This is also seen in almost 100% of patients with doxorubicin. Cardiac toxicities from the latter are not uncommon if the cumulative dose of $400\,\mathrm{mg/m^2}$ is exceeded. For those patients receiving chemotherapy who are premenopausal, about two-thirds will become amenorrheic as a consequence of chemotherapy. Thus, they will in essence also be receiving some hormonal manipulation. However, most women younger than 30 years continue to menstruate during

and after chemotherapy. This holds true for CMF, AC and FAC.

With chemotherapy there has been no evidence of an increased risk of secondary solid tumors; however, myelodysplastic syndrome and acute leukemia occur in greater frequency in the chemotherapy treated population.

MONOCLONAL ANTIBODY DIRECTED THERAPY ± HYPERCALCEMIA

Herceptin, a new form of palliative therapy, is a monoclonal antibody directed against the Her/2 neu surface protein on breast cancer cells. It can interfere with the cell's biological processes and eventually cause cell death. If given with chemotherapy, it may increase the tumor response by 23–32%, and increase the delay in tumor spread by 3 months.

SPECIFIC PALLIATIVE MEDICINE FOR BONE PAIN

Frequently, hormonal manipulation or chemotherapeutic management will control bone pain. If the metastases appear lytic on X-ray, and the pain is not fully controlled with systemic therapy, usually local radiation therapy is considered. When painful areas are multiple, despite chemotherapy or hormonal therapy, Aredia® (Ciba Geneva Pharmaceuticals, Ciba-Geigy Corp., NJ, USA) (pamidronate), a bisphosphonate, that was originally described for hypercalcemia, may be tried. It has recently been approved by the FDA for painful bony metastases as it was found to be efficacious. The use of Aredia and narcotics may mask symptoms or an impending epidural metastasis. Early consultation with a radiation oncologist may avoid the need for emergency surgical or radiation decompression.

RADIATION THERAPY

When a weight-bearing bone has cortical involvement or the spine is collapsing or threatening compression of the spinal cord, local XRT in doses usually 3000–4000 cGy is required. It is effective in pain relief in 73–96% of treated patients. For some situations, up to 5000 cGy may be necessary. Bones that are threatening fracture may need to have internal pins prior to radiotherapy. If facture has occurred, the bone should be treated with radiotherapy to instigate union of the parts. As long as radiation does not have to be delivered over the gastrointestinal tract, 300 cGy/fraction for 10 treatment days in a 2–3 week period is the most cost-effective. If, however, treatment is administered over intestine, stomach, or liver, 150–200 cGy per fraction is suggested to diminish the radiation side-effects.

Palliation for symptoms of pain, shortness of breath, cough, bleeding, neurologic deficit, etc. can be anticipated with a high probability. If radiation is administered simultaneously with hormonal or chemotherapeutic regimens, it is usually reasonably well tolerated.

Radiation also may be used to decompress airway obstruction by tumor, stop bleeding due to tumor, or decrease neurologic compromise.

Few drugs cross the blood–brain barrier. Thus, radiation is commonly used for brain metastasis, whether single or multiple. Often post-surgical removal of a solitary metastasis treatment is given to prevent recurrence. This combination of surgery and radiotherapy seems to increase the chance for long-term survival. If radiation is used alone, an average of only several months survival is reported. There are some long-term survivors, i.e. more than one or two years. Recently, stereotactic radiotherapy or the use of small pencil beams stereotactically positioned with the patient fixed in the CT frame (Gamma Knife), has been employed with promising results equivalent to the combination of surgery and radiation therapy.

Uncommon sites of metastasis may be treated successfully with radiation. Examples are orbital and retinal metastasis. Tumors metastatic to tissues surrounding nerves such as the brachial or sacral plexus causing severe pain may also be relieved by prudent radiotherapy

portals. When there is widespread metastasis, hemibody radiation has successfully reduced pain.

Some palliation can be achieved for widespread bone metastasis with radioactive strontium (^{89}Sr). ^{89}Sr may be used for metastatic bone disease, but frequently causes low platelet counts for prolonged periods of time. Also samarium (^{153}Sa) is available for similar use. Experimentally, rhenium (^{186}Re) is being investigated for similar use.

It must be remembered that metastatic breast disease may continue for very long periods of time, i.e. several years (see Chapter 16). Some patients with widespread metastasis survive for up to 15–20 years. With this knowledge, all forms of therapy must be considered for their long-term sequelae.

Side-effects of radiation therapy

Side-effects of radiation are usually related to the zone of the structures that are included in the radiation portal. For example, if pelvic bones require treatment, the bowel gets in the field requiring irradiation and diarrhea may ensue after several days of treatment. In order for ribs or vertebrae to be treated, the stomach might not be excluded from the exit dose of the field of radiation, thus nausea may occur. These symptoms are usually short-lived and self-limited, disappearing shortly after the therapy has been completed.

HOSPICE

Hospices are currently available throughout the USA and many places in Europe. Patients who do not wish aggressive therapy or who have failed all therapy should take advantage of hospice services. Pain control, daily care, and psychological support may be provided. Most major hospitals are associated with programs which can provide an explanation of their services, appropriate phone numbers, and consultation.

Bibliography

Auchter RM, Lamond JP, Alexander E, *et al.* A multiinstitutional outcome and prognostic factor analysis of radiosurgery for resectable single brain metastasis. *Int J Radiat Oncol Biol Phys* 1996;35: 27–35

Cancer Fax (National Cancer Institute Cancer Data Base) Information from PDQ For Health Professionals. Brain Metastases. *PDQ* 208/03854, 6/98

Christakis NA, Escarce JJ. Survival of medicare patients after enrollment in hospice programs. *N Engl J Med* 1996;172–8

Devita VT, Hellman S, Rosenberg SA. *Cancer Principles and Practice of Oncology*, 4th edn. Philadelphia: J.B. Lippincott Co., 1993

Harris JR, Lippman ME, Morrow M, *et al. Diseases of the Breast.* Philadelphia: J.B. Lippincott Co., 1996

Hortobagyi GN. Progress in endocrine therapy for breast carcinoma. *Cancer* 1998;83:1–6

Moore PM, Kinne DW. The surgical management of primary invasive breast cancer. *CA A Cancer J Clin* 1995;45:279–88

Perez CA, Brady LW. *Principles and Practice of Radiation Oncology*, 2nd edn. Philadelphia: J.B. Lippincott Co., 1992

Breast reconstruction

18

L. Jardines and M. Granick

The widespread use of breast reconstruction after mastectomy began in the 1970s and has continued to gain popularity. It has become an integral part of treatment planning for women with breast cancer. There have been continued advances in the materials and techniques used in breast reconstruction and the cosmetic outcomes continue to improve.

Breast reconstruction after mastectomy makes a difference in a woman whose self-image changes with the alterations in her body that result from the ablative surgery. The plastic surgeon should be part of the health care team which plans the optimal treatment for a woman with breast cancer. The team includes a representative from surgical oncology, radiation therapy, medical oncology, plastic surgery, radiology, pathology, psychiatry, social service and nursing. It is also extremely important that the family physician be involved in the decision-making process since (s)he is often the member of the health care team who knows the patient and the family the best. The reconstruction often consists of a series of stages and must be coordinated among all of the treating physicians.

TIMING OF RECONSTRUCTION

Breast reconstruction can be performed immediately at the time of mastectomy or it can be delayed until adjuvant therapy has been delivered. Initially, there were concerns regarding immediate reconstruction, including the possibility that silicone implants were tumor promoters, and the lengthened surgical time and anesthesia would have an unfavorable effect on the patient's immune system. Other concerns included that it may be difficult to detect a local recurrence after reconstruction and that there may be seeding of tumor in surgical planes developed during the course of the reconstructive procedure. None of these concerns has been substantiated.

There are important advantages to immediate reconstruction which are both psychological and technical. From a psychological standpoint, the patient is far more likely to perceive the reconstruction as a new rather than a mock breast. Technically, the most important landmark is the inframammary fold when performing a breast reconstruction. When the reconstruction is performed immediately, this landmark is still present and the cosmetic outcome is superior. With a delayed reconstruction, this important landmark is obliterated by scar and is difficult to recreate.

Patients with large tumors or palpable axillary nodes may not be optimal candidates for immediate reconstruction, since they are at the highest risk for local/regional recurrence. They will clearly need adjuvant systemic therapy and most likely will require adjuvant chest wall irradiation. A complication associated with the reconstruction may delay the institution of these therapies. In addition, the delivery of adjuvant chest wall irradiation is more complex when the patient has undergone breast reconstruction.

Delayed reconstruction can be performed at any time after the mastectomy; however, there are significant down-sides to performing a late reconstruction. Scarring interferes with the pliability of the skin flaps, which affects the ability to redefine the ablative surgical defect. Many patients are discouraged when it comes to pursuing a delayed breast reconstruction, since it is a second major surgical procedure requiring a second hospitalization and recuperation period, and they never go on to have the surgery. If the patient has received adjuvant chest wall irradiation, there is an increased risk of poor wound healing after the reconstruction. While a good outcome is possible with a delayed reconstruction, an immediate procedure is far more likely to have a positive patient acceptance and appearance.

TYPES OF RECONSTRUCTION

Breast implants and tissue expanders

Until the mid-1970s, the most common technique for breast reconstruction was a breast implant. The outcome is best if the implant is placed in a pocket below the pectoralis major muscle as opposed to the subcutaneous space. The advantages to this procedure is that it adds very little to the operative time, can generally be done as a one-stage procedure and the cost is not high. The cosmetic outcome is generally best in women with small breasts, since it is difficult to attain ptosis in the reconstructed breast (Figure 18.1).

Tissue expanders can be placed in the subpectoral position at the time of mastectomy. The woman returns to the office where saline is added to the reservoir by injecting saline into a special port. The tissue expander is inflated gradually with saline, which allows for a step-by-step stretching of the tissues over time. After a period of 3–4 months, when the tissues have been expanded sufficiently, the expander is removed at a second operation and a permanent implant is placed. With the stretching of the tissues, a larger breast implant can be placed and therefore this technique can be used in women with moderate size breasts (Figure 18.2).

Expansion devices are available which can serve as both the expander and implant. The reservoir is biluminal and contains saline and silicone compartments. When the tissues have

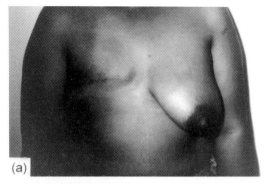

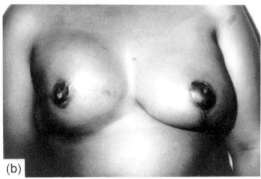

Figure 18.1 (a) Status post-right mastectomy. (b) Status post-right breast reconstruction with a silicone implant and a left mastopexy

been sufficiently expanded, some of the saline is withdrawn from the receiver so that the reconstructed and contralateral breasts are symmetrical. The port used to introduce the saline into the reservoir can be removed as an outpatient surgical procedure.

The advantages and disadvantages of tissue expanders with implants are similar to those of implants alone. Patient selection for the use of either breast implants alone or in conjunction with prior tissue expansion is important. Complications of implants include infection, exposure of the implant and deflation of the expander. Other disadvantages include the development of capsular contracture and rupture or leakage of the implant. The question as to whether silicone in breast implants has been associated with autoimmune diseases was so heavily popularized by the media that it is always a concern to patients. There are many studies which have demonstrated that there is no causal relationship between the presence of silicone implants and autoimmune disease. In addition, breast implants and tissue expanders generally should not be used in women who have had radiation therapy due to the effects of radiation on the skin and soft tissues. Patients who are obese with large ptotic breasts are less likely to have a satisfactory outcome with this method of reconstruction because of the difficulty in achieving symmetry.

Flap procedures

Latissimus dorsi myocutaneous flap

The latissimus dorsi myocutaneous flap was first used for breast reconstruction in 1977. Skin, fat and muscle are rotated from the back to the chest wall and is useful for women who are thin or have had prior abdominal surgery and are not candidates for a transverse rectus abdominus myocutaneous (TRAM) flap. It can also be used for breast reconstruction in women who have received radiation therapy. This flap is not bulky and in many instances, an implant is necessary to provide the needed volume for a breast reconstruction. The latissimus dorsi flap can be extended to include additional subcutaneous tissue such that an implant is not necessary to provide the necessary tissue volume. However, this process may be associated with a higher complication rate, particularly at the donor site. Overall, it is a safe procedure and the flap is extremely reliable.

There does not seem to be a significant functional deficit at the shoulder after the flap has been rotated, although the potential exists. The likelihood of complete flap necrosis is approximately 1% and partial flap necrosis is approximately 5%. The most common complication is at the donor site where the incidence of seroma formation is 10–30%. Among patients in whom an implant is used in conjunction with the flap, the incidence of capsular contracture is between 20 and 50%. Another disadvantage is the resulting scar at the donor site which may be

more visible than the sites of other commonly used flaps. Finally, the flap tends to retract superiorly with the normal healing process causing a late deformity.

Transverse rectus myocutaneous (TRAM) flap

The TRAM was introduced in 1982 and it is the most widely used flap for autologous breast reconstruction. Skin and subcutaneous tissue are harvested through an elliptical incision from the lower abdomen based upon the rectus abdominus muscle which contains the vascular supply via the superior epigastric artery. The flap is then tunneled superiorly through the upper abdominal wall and rotated to the site of the mastectomy defect. The TRAM flap can be based on one or both bellies (single pedicle or bipedicle) of the rectus muscle. The flap provides a large amount of tissue and an implant is rarely needed to provide additional volume, resulting in a natural-appearing and soft reconstructed breast which can have ptosis (Figure 18.3). Another advantage is that the donor scar is transverse in the lower abdomen which can be hidden. In addition, the patient has excess skin and fat removed from the lower abdomen which functions as an abdominoplasty ('tummy tuck').

Recently, the concept of performing a skin-sparing mastectomy in association with immediate breast reconstruction has been reported in the literature. The mastectomy is performed through a keyhole incision to include the nipple and areola; however, the majority of the skin on the chest wall is not excised as with a standard modified radical mastectomy. This leaves a skin envelope into which the tissue from the TRAM flap is placed, avoiding the problem with differing skin tone between the chest and abdominal wall (Figure 18.4).

This flap procedure is a more complex surgical procedure and generally requires 5–7 day hospitalization and 4–6 week recuperation periods. A thorough preoperative evaluation is necessary to select appropriate candidates for the procedure and to reduce the risk of complications. The overall complication rate for the

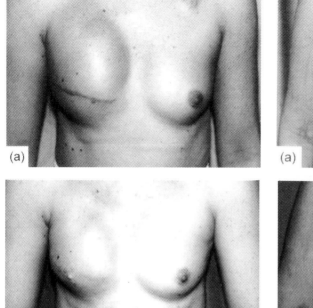

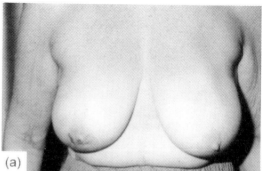

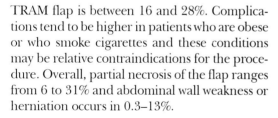

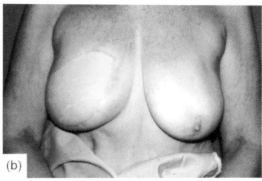

Figure 18.2 (a) Inflated tissue expander in breast pocket. (b) Expander replaced with a permanent implant

Figure 18.3 (a) Preoperative photograph after a right breast biopsy. (b) Ptotic breast after right mastectomy and TRAM flap reconstruction. Note the abdominal skin patch on the reconstructed right breast

TRAM flap is between 16 and 28%. Complications tend to be higher in patients who are obese or who smoke cigarettes and these conditions may be relative contraindications for the procedure. Overall, partial necrosis of the flap ranges from 6 to 31% and abdominal wall weakness or herniation occurs in 0.3–13%.

Free flaps

When a free flap is performed, the tissue is harvested from the donor site and transferred to the defect where a microvascular anastomosis is performed to reconstitute arterial blood supply and venous drainage. The free TRAM flap has been utilized for patients who are thin or have abdominal scars which preclude them from being candidates for a rotational TRAM flap. The vascular supply is based from the inferior epigas-

tric vessels. The vascularity of the tissues with a free TRAM flap is better and a smaller amount of muscle is harvested from the lower abdomen which is associated with lower rates of partial flap slough and abdominal wall complications. The free TRAM flap requires that the plastic surgeon have microvascular surgery expertise and there is always the potential for total flap loss; however, this risk seems to be very small.

Patients who are not candidates for other types of breast reconstruction may be candidates for a free gluteal flap, which was introduced in 1975 and refined in 1983. A portion of the gluteus maximus muscle along with overlying skin based upon either the inferior or superior gluteal vessels is harvested. Concerns with this type of reconstruction include donor site morbidity which includes a potential alteration in hip function. The microvascular

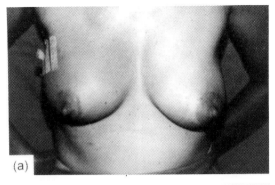

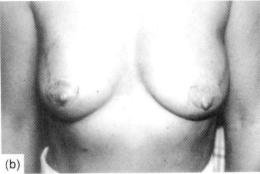

Figure 18.4 (a) Preoperative view of breasts before surgery. (b) Postoperative view after bilateral skin sparing mastectomies and bilateral buried TRAM flaps, nipple reconstructions and areolar tattoos

anastomosis is technically more difficult as well since the vascular pedicle length is shorter.

Breast reconstruction after ipsilateral breast tumor recurrence

The recommended treatment for an ipsilateral breast tumor recurrence when there is no evidence of distant metastasis after lumpectomy and breast irradiation for breast cancer is mastectomy. Many women faced with this situation are interested in breast reconstruction; however, radiation leads to fibrosis, endarteritis and ultimately impaired wound healing. Therefore, patients who have been treated with breast conservation have limited options with respect to reconstruction and are not candidates for implants or tissue expanders. Women who have had prior breast irradiation are also at a higher risk for complications when a TRAM flap is used. Therefore, patients who require mastectomy after an isolated local failure must be carefully evaluated prior to proceeding with breast reconstruction to minimize the likelihood of complications.

Breast reconstruction of the contralateral breast

If the patient already has undergone a mastectomy and a unilateral TRAM flap, this option is no longer available to reconstruct the contralateral breast should mastectomy be the recommended local treatment. In addition, it is often difficult to attain symmetry when a different reconstructive technique is used to reconstruct the ipsilateral and contralateral breasts. It is technically easier for the surgeon and may be emotionally easier for the patient to consider bilateral mastectomies with simultaneous bilateral TRAM flap reconstruction rather than staged ablative surgery and reconstruction. Consequently, patients who are opting for mastectomy with immediate reconstruction to treat the ipsilateral breast and are at high risk for developing a contralateral breast cancer should consider the option of prophylactic contralateral mastectomy with simultaneous bilateral breast reconstruction.

Reconstruction of the nipple and areola

Reconstruction of the nipple and areola is generally delayed until the breast mound reconstruction has had time to heal and mature. Considerable change occurs during the first 3 months after the surgery. As the swelling decreases and gravity affects the tissues, the breast mound actually improves in appearance. After these changes occur, it is appropriate to reconstruct the nipple to match the contralateral side. It is difficult to correct a poorly placed nipple and such an occurrence can undo an otherwise excellent result.

Nipple reconstruction has undergone an evolution during the past 20 years. Initially the nipple was recreated by composite grafting of

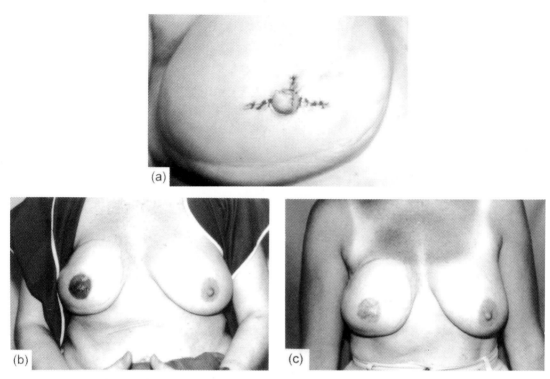

Figure 18.5 (a) The nipple is reconstructed with local skin flaps. (b) The areola is colored with an intradermal tattoo. (c) The color of the tattooed pigment fades over time to match the native areola

an earlobe, toe pad or contralateral nipple. Silicone nipple implants were also used. Currently, a variety of local skin flaps are utilized to obtain nipple projection using the underlying subcutaneous fat for fullness. The areolar repair has similarly undergone changes during the last two decades. Initially, full thickness skin grafts of darker inner thigh skin were used. The method most commonly used now to provide coloration of the skin in areolar reconstruction is intradermal tattooing (Figure 18.5).

Bibliography

Carlson GW. Breast reconstruction. Surgical options and patient selection. *Cancer* 1994;74:436–9

Carlson GW. Skin sparing mastectomy: anatomic and technical considerations. *Am Surgeon* 1996;62:151–5

Corral CJ, Mustoe TA. Controversy in breast reconstruction. *Surg Clin N Am* 1996;76:309–26

Vasconez HC, Holley DT. Use of the TRAM and latissimus dorsi flaps in autogenous breast reconstruction. *Clinics in Plastic Surgery* 1995;22:153–66

Wickman M. Breast reconstruction – past achievements, current status and future goals. *Scand J Plast Reconstr Hand Surg* 1995;29:81–104

Williams JK, Bostwick III J, Breid JT, *et al.* TRAM flap reconstruction after radiation therapy. *Ann Surg* 1995;221:756–66

Epidemiology, genetics and psychosocial aspects of breast disease

19

B.A. Eskin

Breast cancer is a serious threat to women of all ages. During the reproductive years, the breasts may be utilized for nursing. They are specifically affected by hormones from the central nervous system, anterior and posterior lobes of the pituitary, and the ovary. During this period, the breast is a sensitive endocrine target organ which is affected additionally by several endocrine secretions such as thyroid/iodine, insulin and cortisone but basically by estrogens, progesterone and prolactin (Chapter 2). Postpartum and during nursing, oxytocin and probably vasopressin have an influence on the breasts.

In women, breast cancer cases rise linearly through ages 40–70 years but become most prominent in the 'transitional' woman (36 to menopause) (Table 19.1). In menopause, mortality is relatively lower and fewer malignant disease patterns are seen. Several studies indicate that menopausal women on estrogen replacement are still at low mortality.

The female breast is extremely well vascularized as any surgeon appreciates, and typically is affected by fat metabolism, resulting in changes in size and shape. Besides endocrine and metabolic activities, human mammary glands are persistently manipulated by brassières, plastic surgeons and most exercising mechanisms. Because of these multiple intrusions, it is not surprising that breast atypia and neoplasia are potential occurrences throughout a woman's life.

INCIDENCE OF BREAST CANCER

As the decade began, cancer incidence reports (1991) showed that breast cancer led all other cancer sites for women. The American Cancer Society statistics for breast cancer in women during the last 5 years have been about 30% of the total cancer rates, although lung cancer is increasing. Approximately 14% of all women will be subject to neoplasia of the breast in the United States, which is a high-risk region. While breast cancer morbidity has increased, the death rate from breast cancer remains remarkably stable, resulting in a net increase, while 1996 shows a minimal net decrease.

Cancer mortality is a major health problem facing today's industrialized society. Since 1995, breast cancer has fallen to the second leading cause of cancer-related death, but the age-adjusted breast cancer rate remains about the same today as it was 60 years ago. It is estimated that in 1996, 184 300 women were diagnosed with breast cancer and that 44 300 died of the disease. The 5-year relative survival rate now stands at 76%, but for many the surviving years are marred by varying degrees of distress or disability (Figure 19.1).

RISK FACTORS

While almost daily statistical evidence of new risk factors is presented in news broadcasts, its accuracy and relevance seems vague. However,

Table 19.1 Number of deaths from breast cancer* and age-adjusted death rate[†], by state and race[§] – United States, 1988–1992

State	Number of deaths			Rate			Black-to-white ratio
	White	Black	Total	White	Black	Total	
Alabama	2 440	871	3 318	23.5[¶]	31.5	25.2	1.3
Alaska	158	**	190	26.3	**	23.6	**
Arizona	2 609	**	2 707	24.6	**	24.0[¶]	**
Arkansas	1 668	298	1 972	22.9[¶]	30.3	23.8[¶]	1.3
California	18 702	1 579	21 121	26.9	32.1	26.0[¶]	1.2
Colorado	2 169	**	2 260	24.9	**	24.7	**
Connecticut	2 897	181	3 089	26.7	30.0	26.9	1.1
Delaware	593	**	692	32.0	**	32.5	**
District of Columbia	197	509	712	29.3	38.0	35.3[¶]	1.3
Florida	11 859	1 158	13 044	25.2[¶]	29.0	25.5[¶]	1.2
Georgia	3 419	1 116	4 547	24.3[¶]	27.4	24.9[¶]	1.1
Hawaii	177	**	546	25.4	**	18.2[¶]	**
Idaho	712	**	717	25.0	**	24.7	**
Illinois	9 457	1 353	10 853	29.3[¶]	32.8	29.5[¶]	1.1
Indiana	4 513	365	4 888	26.7	33.9	27.2	1.3
Iowa	2 726	**	2 756	26.5	**	26.4	**
Kansas	2 078	**	2 191	25.7	**	25.8	**
Kentucky	2 823	231	3 062	25.4	33.0	25.8	1.3
Louisiana	2 324	1 046	3 386	25.0	33.2	27.2	1.3
Maine	1 110	**	1 116	26.7	**	26.7	**
Maryland	3 188	859	4 073	28.0	32.0	28.6	1.1
Massachusetts	6 110	201	6 335	30.1	31.2	30.0[¶]	1.0
Michigan	6 959	1 071	8 070	27.5	33.7	28.1	1.2
Minnesota	3 686	**	3 744	27.1	**	26.9	**
Mississippi	1 290	631	1 922	22.7	27.8	24.2[¶]	1.2
Missouri	4 271	449	4 734	26.1	32.0	26.6	1.2
Montana	626	**	646	24.8	**	24.8	**
Nebraska	1 431	**	1 463	26.9	**	26.8	**
Nevada	803	**	861	26.7	**	26.3	**
New Hampshire	1 021	**	1 025	30.8	**	30.7	**
New Jersey	7 474	894	8 423	31.5[¶]	34.7	31.6[¶]	1.1
New Mexico	963	**	1 000	24.6	**	23.6	**
New York	16 211	2292	18 643	31.1[¶]	29.6	30.5[¶]	1.0
North Carolina	4 307	1 160	5 518	25.3	30.5	26.3	1.2
North Dakota	564	**	575	27.3	**	27.2	**
Ohio	9404	987	10 409	28.3	32.2	28.6	1.1
Oklahoma	2 259	136	2 468	24.9	24.7	24.0[¶]	1.0
Oregon	2 339	**	2 389	25.7	**	25.4	**
Pennsylvania	12 081	1 089	13 200	29.2[¶]	34.8	29.6[¶]	1.2
Rhode Island	1 103	**	1 141	31.5	**	31.6	**
South Carolina	1 995	745	2 744	25.5	29.0	26.3	1.1
South Dakota	606	**	624	26.5	**	26.3	**
Tennessee	3 358	688	4 056	24.1[¶]	34.2	25.4	1.4
Texas	9 638	1 412	11 100	23.5[¶]	30.3	24.0[¶]	1.3
Utah	883	**	897	23.3	**	23.2	**
Vermont	494	**	494	28.0	**	27.9	**
Virginia	4 035	983	5 057	27.2	33.4	27.9	1.2
Washington	3 713	**	3 851	27.1	**	26.5	**
West Virginia	1 564	**	1 631	24.7	**	24.9	**
Wisconsin	4 312	130	4 455	27.3	33.1	27.3	1.2
Wyoming	320	**	324	25.9	**	25.6	**
Total	189 639	23 114	215 039	27.0	31.3	27.1	1.2

*Decedents for which the underlying cause of death was breast cancer (*International Classification of Diseases, Adapted, Ninth Revision*, codes 174.0–174.9) were identified from public-use mortality data tapes (4).

[†]Per 100 000 women. Adjusted to the age distribution of the 1970 US population.

[§]Numbers for racial/ethnic groups other than black and white were too small for meaningful analysis. However, all totals include numbers for other races.

[¶]The difference between the state-specific rate and the corresponding US rate is statistically significant (p ≤0.0002, Bonferroni-adjusted)

**These data were excluded because the annual average number of persons in the denominator was <75 000.

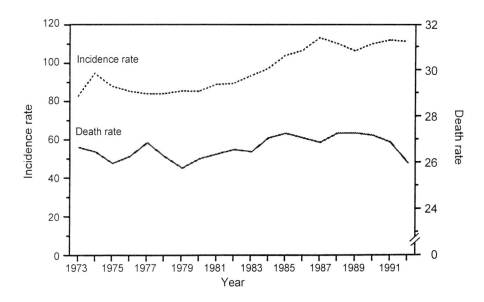

Figure 19.1 Age-adjusted incidence and death rates* for invasive breast cancer[†] – United States, 1973–1992.*Per 100 000 women. Standardized to the age distribution of the 1970 US population. [†]Cases of invasive breast cancer (*International Classification of Diseases, for Oncology*, codes C50.0–C50.9) were registered in SEER. Decedents for which the underlying cause of death was breast cancer (*International Classification of Disease, Adapted, Ninth Revision*, codes 174.0–174.9) were identified from public-use mortality data tapes (4). Source: National Cancer Institute's Surveillance, Epidemiology, and End Results program

for many years the Center for Disease Control and Prevention in Atlanta, Georgia has garnered long-term studies that appear to be consistent.

Family history is essential in establishing risk levels for breast cancer. First-degree relatives of breast cancer patients carry a two- to three-fold increased risk of developing breast cancer. If the cancer relative was premenopausal and had bilateral disease, the risk increases. Risk for the other breast increases when one breast is cancerous, while cancers of the ovary and endometrium also increase the risk. The utilization of gene localization in high-risk families has shown remarkably skewed levels of breast cancer-1 and breast cancer-2 variability in development of the disease. Associations with ovarian and uterine tumors have been recognized.

Conditions which appear to increase breast cancer risk are: early menarche (before 11), late menopause (after 50) and first term pregnancy after 30. Reduction in risk has been attributed to: nursing, full-term pregnancies, oophorectomy before 30.

Obesity is a risk for menopausal women, while it appears unrelated in the premenopause. This may correlate with the socioeconomic risk which increases in the higher strata. Basic concepts become somewhat unclear when these groups are compared considering diet and medical care. High fat diets are involved in peripheral estrone (a reproductive hormone) metabolism, which may be considered precancerous in postmenopausal women while it has no effect on premenopausal women. Intake of coffee (caffeine), tea, methylxanthine foods and beverages, and alcohol (greater than 3 oz/90 g per week) seems to increase the risk. Arguments pro and con have been leveled and all described appear to be difficult to assess.

Whether benign disease is a precursor to breast cancer remains a controversial topic, despite numerous studies. Women with fibrocystic disease were considered originally to have a risk factor four times greater than those without. A study from a committee of the American Pathology Association noted that the risk factor level could only be presented when histopathology was available for diagnosis. Twenty-six per cent of women with proliferative breast nodules are rated at risk. The rating increases if any of the previously described risk factors are also present. About 30% of the risk category have atypical hyperplasia (adenomatous tissue type), which places these individuals at high risk. Atypical hyperplasia, seen on biopsy, on both pre- and postmenopausal women, shows a significant increase in breast cancer.

From these facts, it becomes apparent that a clinical classification is needed which may provide the physician with better criteria for selecting which borderline patients should be biopsied. Some considerations of this dilemma are presented in Table 10.1.

GENETICS AS A RISK FACTOR

In 1994, geneticists announced that they had found and begun mapping two genes that appeared to have responsibility for most cases of inherited breast cancer. The potential for evaluating the risk factor for breasts appeared to be attainable by scanning a woman's genetic pattern. Since that time, many women have sought and obtained serum genetic evaluations in the United States where there was a family history of breast cancer. In this group, 20% underwent prophylactic mastectomies when the gene tested positive, an action that may have been premature.

These genes, named *BRCA1* and *BRCA2* appeared to be associated with reproductive cancer growth in women. It was initially stated that either *BRCA* gene mutation had an 85% risk of developing breast cancer and 60% risk for ovarian cancer. However, a series of recent papers have since shown these levels to be overstated. In 1997, it was reported that over 2% of Ashkenazi Jews carry mutations in *BRCA1* and *BRCA2* that confer increased risks of breast, ovarian and prostate cancer. Evidence from repeat studies showed that the original research was skewed because these studies had been done on women from families where there had been breast cancer. Among women with breast cancer and a family history of the disease, the percentage with *BRCA1* coding-region mutations is less than the 45% predicted by genetic linkage analysis. These results suggest that even in a referral clinic specializing in screening women from high-risk families, the majority of tests for *BRCA1* mutations will be negative and therefore uninformative.

Further research has shown that there are more than 200 potential mutations on each gene and the gene responses vary in young women as compared with menopausal women. Germ-line mutations in the *BRCA2* contribute to fewer cases of breast cancer among young women than do mutations in *BRCA1*. Carriers of *BRCA2* mutations may have a smaller increase in the risk of early-onset breast cancer.

Effectiveness predicated on gene mutations continues to require clarification. Gene mutations may serve as a means of risk assessment with other hereditary factors. Ethnic problems and prophylactic methods are being evaluated.

ESTROGEN AS A RISK FACTOR

Menopausal women are concerned with the effect of replacement estrogen on the breast. This entire issue is clouded by the oral contraceptive controversy as well as the relationship of estrogen to breast cancer etiology. The level of estrogen (usually ethinyl estradiol) given in birth control hormones has estrogen receptor effectiveness approximately seven times the dose used for replacement therapy. When breast cancers are estrogen-dependent as indicated by estrogen and progesterone receptor tumor tissue testing, replacement medication is contraindicated. Except for those specific cancer patients, there appears to be no established contraindication against giving estrogen to women in the menopause for their symptomatology.

No significant increase in risk was shown in a series of relatively acute studies (1–5 years) as well as persistent therapy over 12 years in menopausal women. Latency series (15–20 years) similarly have not resulted in breast changes that can significantly change the longevity or comfort of the patient. Ongoing studies are continuing in women who are over 70 years and on estrogen replacement since responses in late menopause (over 65 years) have not yet been fully evaluated. Early data show a mild rise in risk for this group which is considered insignificant in light of the cardiovascular and bone protection afforded by estrogen.

When risk factor observation of birth control steroids is used, there have been evident vacillations of results. The Cancer and Steroid Hormone Study (CASH) and the Center for Disease Control evaluated almost 5000 cases of breast cancer (ages 20–45 years) seeking confirmation of whether there is an increased risk with birth control pills. Most recent studies from these groups and others have shown no significant differences even using age of first utilization data. The research continues considering several other related reproductive factors as well. Considering the remarkably reduced estrogen level used in estrogen replacement (1:7), these results bode well for estrogen use.

Progesterone therapy is recommended to be taken with estrogen replacement whenever the patient has a uterus. In menopausal women, unopposed estrogen therapy causes the endometrium to be activated and may result in atypia, which may cause endometrial neoplasia. Whether progesterone is essential similarly when estrogen is given alone to protect the breast tissues remains indefinite. The American Society for Reproductive Medicine has stated that it is unnecessary on the basis of available evidence to add progesterone cyclically for breast protection in replacement therapy.

Biochemically, estrogen metabolism can be restricted at certain cell levels, mutagenically and receptor-wise. The resulting growth may deviate and become neoplastic in older tissues where several atypical pathways of development are described. Some forms of progesterone, such as medroxyprogesterone acetate and megestrol acetate, have been shown to lower the general risk when given simultaneously. In individuals with high risk of the genes for breast cancer, the use of progesterone has not changed the increasing risk seen after 15 years of estrogen therapy when compared to those women without risk.

PSYCHOSOCIAL ASPECTS OF BREAST DISEASE

Many vivid media accounts of women's encounters with breast cancer have raised intense public awareness of how trying such an experience can be. Such concerns are reflected in the abundant and growing literature on breast cancer and psychosocial factors. Psychosocial factors relate to diagnosis, treatment, rehabilitation, and maintenance, and, when necessary, terminal care. They also operate in early stages of the disease, before it is detected, and at the time of detection.

The psychologic and sociologic implications of breast disease seem to be separate issues. Psychologically, the threat of death overwhelms the patient, while the social complexity of body disfigurement remains extant. This chapter will discuss the psychologic and sociologic factors separately, but will eventually combine these elements. The presently accepted solutions will be described, but exhaustive accounts can be found in referenced texts.

Distress syndrome

Every physician involved in the case should accept the responsibility of following the patient through all the stages of diagnosis and post-cancer maintenance. The need for serious psychosocial consideration and sympathetic attitude remain uppermost throughout. The attention to detail in obtaining information is often lost to the patient, due to the emotional state involved. It is important, first, that one provider be identified who will responsibly inform the patient of the overall status. This individual should be trusted by the patient for data sorting and questions that develop. This interested physician should serve as the facilitator of all the information that evolves for the patient. This should be the primary physician (internist, generalist, obstetrician/gynecologist), or later on, the oncologist, radiotherapist, chemotherapist, surgeon, psychologist, psychiatrist – running through the entire hierarchy of involved physicians. Regardless, the established individual responsible for informing and explaining all the basic factors maintains that position. The specialists should add to the picture by detailing their expertise. The cornerstone factors of a good facilitator are:

(1) Information.
(2) Trust.
(3) Support.
(4) Anticipation.
(5) Interaction.
(6) Responsibility.
(7) Providing adequate second opinion opportunities.

Periods of distress

Prediagnostic

When a patient is diagnosed as having breast cancer, several writers feel there is an insatiable desire to obtain 'knowledge and the sense of empowerment' that this may afford. Patients have been known to spend copious time in libraries and other medical informational sources. Especially effective are the web sites and computer-based search modalities such as MEDLINE. Often the patient may join support groups and spend a great deal of conversation time with women who have undergone similar problems. These packets of information from several sources permit her to arrive at decisions that may not be in keeping with those the breast specialist may have suggested. Psychosocial pressures may overcome medical logic. If a friend or relative has done well with certain therapies, the subtleties of practice may be

disregarded. This calls for logical handling and careful consideration of the woman's emotional status. Consider the alternatives and use the information available to explain carefully the values you consider most important. Many patients blame physicians for not offering this service.

Early diagnostic phase

Whether found on self-examination, by the physician, or by mammography, the awareness of a breast lump will strike terror in a woman. This fear may overwhelm all consults and conferences that mean to instruct her. The style of the doctor–patient relationship established during the work-up greatly influences the outcome of the psychologic and social issues that generally arise. This needs to be kept uppermost in the minds of the care givers if cooperation and a constructive doctor–patient team are to be created.

The more expeditious and efficient a breast lump work-up is, the better for the patient. While waiting for the final word on the benign or malignant nature of the mass, the patient is distraught and further depressed by the worse prognoses which she may imagine. Hopefully she has shared her concerns with a loved one, and he or she is not equally caught up in these fears. The sensitivity of contact individuals such as nursing personnel, the doctor's staff, and social workers towards the fragile psyche of these women may set the tone for the next phase of her care.

The patient needs to feel that she can ask questions – repeatedly if necessary – at all stages of their care and of all care givers. When answering you need to be direct, complete, and without medical jargon. Because the same questions may be asked of several contacts, it is not unusual for patients to hear what seems to them to be conflicting answers. This is extremely disturbing and renders the discussion unreliable. Time spent patiently and lovingly explaining does help. Written information dispensed during the early diagnostic phase can help if it is not too complex. Because the diagnosis is not yet made, this is not the time to use a pamphlet that talks about the fine points of management or the side-effects of chemotherapy. Providing the entire scenario for a not-yet diagnosed serious illness is not useful.

Presenting the diagnosis of breast cancer

Women should ideally hear the dreaded diagnosis of breast cancer in the company of an understanding loved one. Doctors need to schedule plenty of time for tears and to present several options for treatment. Women usually are sufficiently disturbed that the repetition of the information given is essential. When possible a written sheet which carefully explains the care options is helpful and in some states such a disclosure sheet is required by law. Encouraging patients to bring in written questions can improve initial exchanges of information. One technique used is a simple cassette tape recorded during office visits which allows her to review her questions and your answers, and advice at home. This permits her to present this information accurately to other members who are concerned and often initiates a discussion of the facts.

Patients should be informed of how time may be an essential ingredient to success. They may have to make up their minds about care options more quickly than they would like. Most centers show no degradation of outcome with up to a 3-week interval between diagnosis and definitive care. The longer the waiting period, however, the more indecision and confusing anecdotal advice may plague the patient and her family, beyond the medical reality.

While women seem to do better emotionally if they take charge of their care and feel that they can influence that care, most are ill-equipped to make sophisticated clinical decisions. The careful teaching of the anatomy, vocabulary, and options of management are of primary importance in helping women make decisions. A specially trained registered nurse or physician's assistant can help greatly with this education.

Involving the patient in self-education and making her a member of the team that is being marshaled to provide her care is feasible and essential. This involvement will benefit the patient by making her feel empowered and the center of the therapeutic considerations. From this, the doctor will be rewarded with a helpful rather than hindering patient as the complex demands on her mental, physical, and emotional coping skills arise. With this style of care patients feel listened to, cared about, and joined in their struggle.

The time of presentation of the diagnosis is often the time to begin forming a team to provide her care. It is always useful and advantageous to encourage the patient to seek a second opinion as soon as a program is suggested. Many patients are reluctant to ask for a second opinion for fear that it will be read by the treating physician as a lack of confidence or, worse yet, as an insult. Many think that such a presumed slight will negatively affect their care.

The patient and her family should know that everything possible is being done for her physical and emotional well-being. If she is introduced to a radiation oncologist or an oncologist specializing in breast cancer, many questions on her mind may be answered immediately. Some centers provide a registered nurse or social worker who is readily available by phone and specially trained in this field. This can be an invaluable resource to the patient and a major physician time-saver.

Distress reactions with surgery

Breast surgery is both a physical and an emotional assault on feelings of femininity and sexuality. Patients are initially caught up in the basic worry that this illness may lead to death, while simultaneously working out optimal treatment plans with her consultants. It is not until the breast is removed or disfigured that the grief of this loss may express itself fully. Feeling that they have coped well through the surgical phase of care, the patient is surprised to find herself depressed and mourning at a time when she thought the worst was over. The well-known sequence of: (1) denial, (2) anger, and (3) sadness followed by (4) acceptance is often delayed by the use of coping mechanisms developed for the surgery. Later (5) distress often comes several months after diagnosis and initial treatment. It should be anticipated by the doctor and watched for by trained staff or forewarned family members.

A study of the psychosocial responses of women to breast surgery found wide variety in the depth and manifestations of psychosocial problems and particularly in their timing. This study found that women who were emotionally intact and mature prior to surgery did best, as anticipated. On the other hand, those patients who had shown psychological maladaptation to pregnancy, menses, or marriage required more intervention and time. Even the most poised and able women, however, may find the double threats of disfigurement and death daunting prospects. It is incumbent upon the primary care physician, or the doctor who sees the patient and family frequently, to alert the patient of the emotional component of breast cancer and to provide reassurance that she will heal emotionally as well as physically. The patient should be referred to supportive care groups or practitioners as needed.

Evidence of depression may be masked by the patient, who tries to be cheerful and contained. The true nature of the patient's mood will only reveal itself if time is taken to listen in a non-judgmental fashion with an ear attuned to the typical signs and symptoms of depression. The patient first must come to grips with the life-threatening aspects of her diagnosis. Only then can she begin to take other steps necessary to mourn her loss. Every effort should be made to encourage the expression of feelings of anger, sadness, fear, and grief by counseling. Inquiry by knowledgeable individuals and psychiatric or group counseling referrals should be used early if necessary.

Postsurgical psychosocial problems

Except in cases of needle biopsy, women begin the emotional healing process by accepting scarring and local discomfort of the breast after initial tissue biopsies. Postoperatively, the breast is never the same and its appearance will be a constant reminder of her neoplasia to both her and her partner. A scar that looks tiny to the physician always looks larger and more disfiguring to the patient.

The physician's knowledge of how scars age, change, and fade may allow him or her to overlook angry redness or minor lumps that will flatten, and to disregard transient paresthesias. These distortions, however, may be of major concern to the patient. Explanations about the stages of healing and everlasting reassurance avoid later psychological reactions. Several manuals described the error of telling a woman her mastectomy or scar 'looks wonderful' as a poor choice of words at a serious time. Using such an approach will lose her or his relationship with the patient at a time when she needs honest help the most. The expressions 'healing normally' 'doing fine', or 'just like it should be at this stage', often relieve some anxiety with directness. Downplaying the family's revulsion, horror, or fear will not be constructive. Patients and families have a completely different frame of reference than the physician does in this matter. They have probably never seen surgical scarring before. Their minds and bodies are hurting with a result which cannot go away.

Patients and their partners are often frightened or revolted by the appearance of the surgical site. Explaining the shape, texture, and color of the scar during dressing changes helps. Reassurance about normal healing stages every day speeds acceptance.

Breast reconstruction

For some women, breast reconstruction at the time of primary surgery or soon thereafter is essential for emotional rehabilitation. For others prolonged or repeat surgery is anathema. Results of reconstruction, while often excellent, do not produce a mass that feels like or functions as a breast. The value of the reconstructed breast is largely in the eye of the beholder; it may be of great or little importance depending on the individual patient. For some women, how they look to others, especially men, is paramount. Patients need to see photographs of real reconstructions under daily conditions, not just of the best outcomes but typical outcomes as well. Ideally, they should be permitted to speak with other patients who have and have not chosen to undergo a breast reconstruction. After such a session, they should be free to make their own decision.

As described in several women's magazines, a reconstructed breast that looks perfect in clothing may look peculiar in night clothes or in the nude. The actual appearance, texture, and feel of the reconstructed breast may not be pleasing to the patient or her partner. Many women do not realize that it is often obvious to one who casually hugs her that one breast is hard and the other soft, as can happen with some procedures. The loss of erotic sensations in the reconstructed breast may not be a primary issue, but it deserves consideration before surgery so that it may be more readily coped with afterward (see Chapter 18).

While techniques differ, most surgical reconstructions avoid the need for external removable pads and allow the patient to appear clothed as she did prior to surgery. Nevertheless, the latest external, removable prostheses are so lifelike and adaptable that they are fully satisfactory to most older, emotionally stable women. The external prostheses can be glued onto the chest for days at a time or stuffed into a myriad of lacy garments for any and all clothed activities without fear of being dislodged or obviously identified.

Late or delayed postsurgical reactions

Some patients will show no adverse psychological symptoms immediately after mastectomy. This is not usually a healthy sign, although both the patient and doctor wish it were. These delayed reactions manifest themselves several months or years later when major life changes, such as a family death or divorce, rob the patient of her last traces of self-denial, compensatory coping mechanisms or ego strength. The delayed reaction may seem to be unrelated to the breast surgery. The cause of her obscure depression or personality change will be difficult to determine and there may be resistance to both release and psychotherapy. When the cause is extracted, a thorough and intimate discussion of her feelings about the malignancy would be necessary. An in-depth discussion of her personal life would unearth underlying currents of distress. However, it is never easy to ask a patient specific questions about intercourse, petting, nude behavior, or fantasy life. Nevertheless, until such issues are inquired about the patient may be unable to speak of them.

Intimate questions give patients the 'permission' to have these private feelings, to speak about them, and to seek and get answers to questions they dared not ask before. It is not unusual to unearth a great deal of psychosexual dysfunction on the part of the patient or her mate in these interviews. Sometimes problems will surface which had existed earlier and had never been resolved prior to the cancer.

Cancer outcome: personality and social factors

There is a persistence of self-guilt with any illness. This is intensified by general media commentary on the availability of self-help regimens for prevention which was never attainable except by the innovator. A variety of psychological variables have been reported to be associated with breast cancer progression particularly in certain groups. The psychological focus has been placed on social support, helplessness, depression and emotional expression. Data from a number of studies have been noted to affect these factors, both positively and negatively. This is an active research area and the results that have emerged suggest that study in the area of psychological factors and cancer progression may well bear fruit.

Social support

The association between increased social support from significant others and decreased stress has been demonstrated. How strongly this relationship extends to cancer abrogation is not absolutely clear. The evidence from several reports – animal, clinical, and epidemiological – is suggestive but not consistent. Scientifically, there is conflicting evidence from studies and reviews which reflect only the complex nature of this type of research. Large sociologic groups who provide support claim a 25–30% improvement. The weight of the evidence, however, suggests that support enhances both mental and physical health in a variety of populations.

Helplessness and hopelessness: depression

The same kind of conclusions were drawn both for depression as for helplessness-hopelessness. Hopelessness was manifested by scores on a scale of future despair. It appeared to be predictive of important life events and showed significance in predicting the severity of disease. It is possible, under some conditions and tumor modifications, that patients with non-pathological depression have a poorer prognosis than those without such depression. While these subpopulations are hard to designate, some individuals manifested critical changes in the prognosis of their disease. The population subject to increased risk of poor prognosis in the presence of non-pathological depression is limited.

Expression of emotion

Under some conditions, for some patients, poor emotional expression may portend earlier relapse or death. Several authors' conceptualization of risk addresses some of these underlying issues. For example, the physiological mechanisms underlying repressed emotional expression increases host vulnerability. Such mechanisms need to be examined in detail and tested but show a definite direction.

Fighting spirit and aggression

The findings that a 'fighting spirit' was associated with longer survival in stage I and II breast cancer patients has good support. If we can equate the expressed hostility with fighting spirit, this is a salient positive position. Similarly, it was found that uncooperative, feisty, complaining breast cancer patients (all metastatic) survived longer than 'good' patients. Apparently, positive studies on unpleasant patients, and to some extent, those showing inability to express emotion, support one another.

Sexuality

The constant barrage of breast nudity, cleavage, and symmetrical torso curvature on magazine covers, billboards, and movie screens is an acid reminder to the patient of what she has lost. Covert surgical losses of other body parts, such as the colon, lung, or spleen do not elicit these problems, largely because these tissues have less sexual connotation and are not constantly related to sexuality in the public eye. The breast has psychosocial aspects beyond its function which provide a need for the physician to promote total emotional and physical healing.

The postoperative state

After a mastectomy, few husbands or lovers admit to sexual problems due to the disfigurement. During their interviews, most fear that they may cause discomfort or disrupt the healing surgical site. This problem remains generally for only a short time after the recovery period. Most men stated that their erotic satisfaction remained unchanged and could provide the partner with this reassurance. This affirmation is remarkably important as non-breast sexual activity assumes greater importance in the postsurgical patient. The counselor encourages hugs, massages, showering together, and all forms of petting and erotica when acceptable to both partners. The wife senses sexual satisfaction in her partner by physiologic results and persistent or renewed desire. Lack of these conclusive factors leads to serious problems, regardless of his testimony.

Changed libido on the part of the patient or her partner is multifaceted. Disfigurement, discomfort, and depression all contribute to changed sexual responsiveness. The side-effects of adjuvant therapy, fatigue, and depression resulting from radiation treatments may contribute to decreased frequency of intercourse. Adjuvant therapy itself may decrease the female libido. These therapeutics cause a decrease in ovarian response with concomitant reduced secretion of estrogens and other hormones. From the hypoestrogen state vaginal dryness with dyspareunia may result, which leads to intercourse difficulties.

Sexual intercourse

Sexual intercourse should be encouraged as soon as the patient is comfortable. Resumption of this normal activity can be psychosexually therapeutic. Patients may require suggestions for intercourse positions which may be more desirable. Personal experimentation works well, but a recommendation is that the first time might be with the woman on top, that coitus take place in a recliner chair, or in any fashion that early on does not involve the surgical site so that it must bear the full weight of the partner's body. Also suggested, patients in the 'missionary position' can be instructed to place the affected arm across the chest with the hand on the opposite shoulder to create a protective bridge over the surgical site or to cover the surgery with a small pillow until she is without discomfort. Again, you may want to reassure them that normal sexual activity will not cause harm.

Women often will want to wear a light prosthesis with their night clothes until they are comfortable and used to the scarring. Now is the time for treating the patient to new, indulgent sexy lingerie (Victoria's Secret, etc.), preferably bought by or with the spouse or lover.

Few patients or mates will ask the 'When can we?' question. Doctors need to suggest, remind, or even assign sexual intercourse as a healing activity.

Bras and clothing

As soon as the patient is able to dress, simple and inexpensive adjustments can be made to bras and clothing. A symmetrical breast appearance is a tonic to the post-surgical patient. Several authors suggest soft, clean cotton stuffed into a section of old nylon stocking makes a light false breast to place in the bra cavity initially. To prevent discomfort and healing problems in the surgical areas, utilize a sports bra or else the clips that control the length of bra straps should be placed over the back, preferably over the scapulae.

A soft stuffed bra can usually be worn by the tenth postoperative day. Until the vacant bra cup is filled with something, clothing will not drape properly, and patients may be reluctant to be seen in public. Women with modified radical mastectomies or more than 30% removal of breast tissue will need something similar in texture and weight to normal breast tissue to fill the vacant bra cup after full healing has taken place.

Prostheses

Breast reconstruction may serve this purpose (see Chapter 18). In the absence of reconstruction, the primary physician should become knowledgeable about local sources of bras, expert fitters, and prostheses. A phone call to the local American Cancer Society or Mastectomy Support Group can establish where these businesses are located. Surgical supply houses carry prostheses but they are not necessarily equipped to provide a pleasant experience for the patient. Often surrounded by bedpans, wheelchairs, and all manner of replacement parts and sickroom supplies, they tend to become reminiscent of hospital care. Some companies will detail the patient with literature and samples available to feel. Many major urban department stores have a brassière fitter (who may or may not have special training) in the lingerie department, but these stores are usually limited to one brand or style. In large metropolitan areas, boutiques devoted to the unique clothing needs of breast surgical patients, including lingerie, swimwear, and pocketed bras, are appearing, and will often sell by mail order. The fitting of the first postoperative bra and prosthesis is emotionally very taxing and patients should not go alone. Staring at the nude scarred chest is inevitable and brings home the permanence of the deformity.

Bras come with and without pockets. Prostheses are made with and without nipples. Much trial and error in the first 6 months after surgery is needed before a comfortable and attractive fit is obtained. You should advise the patient to buy one bra at a time. Some stores may allow prostheses to be taken on a trial basis. While some insurance plans cover these costs, not all have the same requirements. If the doctor prescribes the prosthesis and the shop receipt notes 'surgical prosthesis', both copies should be made available to support the claim. The prostheses cost about $600, and with normal wear and gentle care lasts 12–18 months. Changes in body weight of about 10 pounds or more necessitate a new garment.

During the 6-week or 3-month postoperative office visit, the surgeon or nurse should discuss these cosmetic needs for the patient. When surgical reconstructions have been done, the active sportswoman must feel secure that her external silicone breast will not shift and embarrass her while jogging, bowling, playing tennis, or any other sport. The newer sports bras may also be purchased with pockets for the prostheses.

Some women prefer to wear their prosthesis in a light lacy bra in bed at night. The larger the remaining breast, the more necessary this is for shoulder comfort. Some authors state that a soft mattress or water bed that conforms to the body and fills in the space left by breast removal makes this practice unnecessary.

Adjuvant therapy and psychological recovery

When adjuvant therapy is prescribed, the treatment of breast cancer illness is drawn out. While some women have few side-effects, most have periods of generalized illnesses secondary to the therapy. Some chemotherapy further complicates body image and self-esteem by causing hair loss. A pretreatment wig fitting can help to ease this transition, with hair pieces designed to mimic the hair before its thinning or loss. Women should be assured that hair will regrow.

Anti-estrogen treatment leads to a condition which mimics the menopause. All the menopausal symptoms, such as skin and breast changes, vaginal dryness and hot flashes, are present. Topical applications of non-estrogenic moisturizers will improve vulvovaginal lubrication while water-soluble lubricants at the time of intercourse are important for ease and comfort. The changes in the breast can change the size of the remaining breast tissue, necessitating refitting of the prosthesis.

The role of the support group

Postmastectomy support groups have grown abundantly. Doctors should try to arrange for a visit to their patients by the special support groups represented in the center or hospital setting during the surgery admission. These groups are usually able to provide the assistance in the patient's locale. These volunteers are women with breast cancer (at least 1 year postoperatively) who bring role-model support, information, and a kit that contains a temporary bra-stuffing form. Ongoing, long-term support groups, especially for those undergoing chemotherapy, are extremely useful. As described previously, an increase in survival time of those attending such a group was presented in one study. Women feel at ease and share hopes, fears, coping mechanisms, and information.

Written material about breast cancer can be obtained from the public library and specialized lay medical libraries. Much is professionally written, while other works are biographical, anecdotal, or simplified. Most patients are helped by extensive reading, but unfortunately, others are frightened; the reading recommendations need to be tailored accordingly.

Referral sources – psychotherapy

When you identify psychological distress as a cause of delay for your patient's recovery, you must decide whether referral is necessary. As a general rule, a patient still in trouble 6 months or more after surgery needs sophisticated and time-consuming help. The cheapest and often the best help comes from breast cancer support groups, which have already been described. If the patient cannot be persuaded to attend an initial meeting or none is available in her community, refer her to a counselor who may specialize in these cases. Because treatment usually consists of allowing the patient to vent her feelings in a safe setting, a clinical psychologist or marriage counselor often does well. Referring the patient to her pastor, rabbi, or other religious figure sometimes can be sufficient, if that is the patient's choice. When the status is upgraded to a neurotic or psychotic level, the use of a psychiatrist or psychiatric clinic becomes necessary.

When there are a variety of treatment decisions for breast cancer and neither the patient nor family members can visualize their needs, a psychotherapist can be helpful. Often the choices of lumpectomy or mastectomy, elective chemotherapy, possible prophylactic mastectomy of the healthy breast, and the option of reconstructive surgery present options that none of the medical team desires specifically to advise. In addition to the actual treatment choices and an overwhelming anxiety about the cancer, the patient is also faced with a number of specialists, which may include an internist or gynecologist, a radiologist or radiotherapist, a breast surgeon, an oncologist, a radiation oncologist, and a plastic surgeon. It is clear that psychological factors affect the appropriateness of patients' decisions and, frequently, their success with treatment.

The use of an individual specially trained in psychotherapy, but knowledgeable in oncology, may be essential and useful to the patient and her family. These individuals address the emotional responses of patients, families, and caretakers (psychosocial) as well as the psychological, social and behavioral factors that may influence cancer morbidity and mortality. Breast cancer patients may find such services available in the hospital, where the medical care is obtained and useful during diagnosis, treatment, and recovery. During the treatment and recovery phases, patients and families need allies who can offer support, initiate psychological interventions, and facilitate assertiveness training. This psychotherapist may be called upon to treat the side-effects of surgery (scars and loss of the breast) and adjuvant treatments (including feelings about hair loss, fatigue, nausea, and vomiting). General anxiety throughout the course of the illness and fears of recurrence are also common presenting symptoms.

The psychotherapist is often helpful in working with the partner, children, and parents of the breast cancer patient. Regardless of the fact that breast cancer is a publicly acknowledged illness, we still find that the families of breast cancer patients may suffer because of their relative obscurity and neglect. The psychological treatment for breast cancer should routinely include interventions for both the patient and family. Interestingly, partners and children will often require support for legitimizing their needs.

Financial stress, transportation needs, and child care arrangements are some of the issues that face the families of breast cancer patients. Frequently, the ambience in the home changes as the healthy spouse assumes his double workload, and the focus of attention is shifted from the children to the sick parent. Neglect and loneliness, both psychological issues, may occur in children of breast cancer patients. These problems can place these children at a serious psychological risk. It is often wise to consult appropriate therapists during the course of the breast surgery and treatment to consider whether family therapy might not be appropriate.

Bibliography

Anderson BC, Kiecolt-Glaser JK, Glaser R. A biobehavioral model of cancer stress and disease course. *Am Psychol* 1994;49:389–404

Coscarelli-Schag CA. Characteristics of women at risk for psychosocial distress in the year after breast cancer. *J Clin Oncol* 1993;11:783–93

Couch FJ, De Shano ML, Blackwood MA, *et al.* BRCA1 mutations in women attending clinics that evaluate the risk of breast cancer. *N Engl J Med* 1997; 336:1409

Fawzi F, Kemeny M, Fawzy N, *et al.* A structured psychiatric intervention for cancer patients. II: Changes over time in immunological measures. *Arch Gen Psychiatry* 1990;47:792–5

Gersh W, Bobbins DM. *Psychological Treatment of Cancer Patients: A Cognitive Behavioral Approach.* Boston: Allyn and Bacon, 1992

Haber (ed). *Breast Cancer – A Psychological Treatment Manual.* New York: Springer Publishing Company, 1995

Kiecolt-Glaser J, Glaser R, Dyer C, *et al.* Chronic stress and immunity in family caregivers of Alzheimer's disease victims. *Psychosom Med* 1987;49: 523–35

Krainer M, Silva-Arrieta S, Fitzgerald MG, *et al.* Differential contributions of BRCA1 and BRCA2 to early-onset breast cancer. *N Engl J Med* 1997;336: 1416–21

MMWR. *Cancer Facts and Figures.* 1996;45: 833–7

Roa BB, Boyd AA, Volcik K, *et al.* Ashkenazi Jewish population frequency for common mutations in BRCA1 and BRCA2. *Nat Genet* 1996;14:185–7

Schain WS, Fetting JH. Modified radical mastectomy versus breast conservation: psychosocial considerations. *Semin Oncol* 1992;19:239–43

Spiegel D, Bloom J, Kraemer H, *et al.* Effect of psychosocial treatment on survival of patients with metastasis breast cancer. *Lancet* 1989;8668:888–91

Struewing JP, Hartge P, Wacholder S, *et al.* The risk of cancer associated with specific mutations of BRCA1 and BRCA2 among Ashkenazi Jews. *N Engl J Med* 1997;336:1401

Follow-up after breast cancer treatment and prevention

20

S.O. Asbell

FOLLOW-UP

In the USA, follow-up after breast cancer treatment has become a major controversial issue since health maintenance organizations began to dictate policy. Recent reviews state that most diagnostic studies to evaluate for metastasis in patients with early stage breast cancer are not cost-effective. Finding tumors earlier when the patient is not symptomatic fails to lengthen survival and in only one study improved the quality of life. Although tests such as carcinoembryonic antigen (CEA), liver enzymes, and chest X-rays have not proven to change the patient's survival, if the patient has known metastases these tests appropriately ordered may help improve the quality of the patient's life by recognizing disease spread or recurrence early enough to avoid irreversible damage. We must not only keep survival and its cost in mind but understand and consider the quality of life that could be effected by not allowing bulky sites of tumor to develop. Sufficient studies evaluating follow-up and quality of life in stage III advanced disease have not yet been completed.

Most agree that if the disease can be controlled locally, the chances for dissemination are less. Thus, early detection of recurrences or disease in the opposite breast with yearly mammography is vital to understanding the local status and thus control of disease. Once a patient has completed radiation therapy after lumpectomy, a baseline study should be performed 6 months later and then yearly. Should there be new microcalcifications suspicious for recurrence or new tumor, the disease may be curtailed while it is still in a curable state. Follow-ups should be at 6-month intervals unless the patient has had known metastatic disease for which more frequent intervals are suggested. Monitoring metastatic disease once present may require frequent X-rays, bone scans, and liver function studies to provide proper quality of care. Common sites of metastases seen at autopsy are noted in Table 20.1.

Late side-effects of radiation and sequelae may not be recognized by the physician unaccustomed to assessing the irradiated breast or metastatic sites. Therefore, the radiation oncologist should participate in regular follow-up. This is particularly important if the patient has received chemotherapy as well. Late effects of combined modality therapy with some of the newer agents have not yet been fully realized.

Good follow-up should include yearly pelvic exams, especially in women receiving hormonal therapy. All patients on hormones who experience extramenstrual bleeding should have a gynecologic examination.

BREAST CANCER PREVENTION

Weight control

There is some evidence that obesity is related to the development of breast cancer. Thus, programs which by diet and exercise assist in weight reduction or the maintenance of appropriate weight may help reduce cancer risk.

157

Table 20.1 Metastases of 167 consecutive autopsied breast carcinoma cases

	Site	%
1.	Lung	77.2
2.	Bone	73.1
3.	Mediastinal nodes	66.5
4.	Pleura	64.7
5.	Liver	61.1
6.	Adrenal	53.9
7.	Abdominal nodes	44.3
8.	Pericardium	35.3
9.	Axillary nodes	32.9
10.	Peritoneum	24.6
11.	Diaphragm	24.6
12.	Ovary	23.4
13.	Breast	21.6
14.	Skin	18.6
15.	Spleen	16.8
16.	Cervical nodes	15.0
17.	Gastrointestinal tract	14.4
18.	Pancreas	13.8
19.	Kidney	12.6
20.	Pituitary	9.0
21.	Heart	8.4
22.	Uterus	8.4
23.	Ureter	7.8
24.	Gallbladder	6.6
25.	Thyroid	5.4
26.	Esophagus	4.2
27.	Fallopian tubes	3.6
28.	Pineal gland	2.4
29.	Inguinal nodes	2.4
30.	Bladder	2.4
31.	Common bile duct	1.8
32.	Vagina	1.2
33.	Trachea	–
34.	Parotid gland	–
35.	Brain (cerebral)(dural)	28.3/33.3
36.	Spinal cord	–

Diet control

Some studies suggest that diets high in fruits and vegetables decrease the risk of breast cancer, although this evidence is much weaker than that for other cancer sites. Some studies relate alcohol consumption with an increased risk of breast cancer. In postmenopausal women on hormonal replacement therapy, increased estradiol levels have been reported following alcohol consumption (up to 327%). Exposure to organochlorines or diets high in fat may also be associated with an increased breast cancer risk.

Chemoprevention

Chemoprevention is the intervention with chemical agents before malignancy (invasion across the epithelial basement membrane) develops, with the objective of halting or slowing carcinogenesis. Currently the most heavily studied agents are tamoxifen and the retinoids. The major strategy of chemoprevention is to block the effects of both epithelial mutagens and mitogens on neoplastic progression. The aims are to modulate specific steps in the carcinogenic process, prevent DNA damage by free radicals, suppress epithelial cell proliferation, and increase epithelial cell differentiation. Because a long period will be required to prevent cancer the agent must be associated with a low rate of clinical toxicity.

It is believed that the high susceptibility of the terminal duct lobular units of the breast to carcinogenic transformation and progression is due to the high proliferative rate of the breast epithelium in these structures. Clearly, both estrogen and progesterone play critical roles in the pathogenesis of breast cancer, at least partly due to their proliferative effects on breast epithelium. While estrogen enhances breast epithelial proliferation, tamoxifen blocks this process and thus is considered a possible chemopreventive agent. A new agent, Raloxifene, is under study.

WHICH CANDIDATES MIGHT BENEFIT THE MOST FROM CHEMOPREVENTION?

Women with a 20% or greater lifetime risk of developing breast cancer including those with genetic predispositions, strong family histories, proliferative breast diseases, and non-invasive cancers, are currently considered good candidates for participating in chemopreventive trials with novel agents. Genetic screening for germline mutations in the *BRCA1* or *BRCA2* gene can be used to predict up to an 85% lifetime risk of developing breast cancer. Women with a strong family history of breast cancer (two first-degree relatives affected or one first-degree and two second-degree relatives affected) or of breast and ovarian cancers (three affected relatives with breast cancer and one relative with ovarian cancer) are also good candidates for chemoprevention, since their lifetime risk of developing breast cancer is 25–30%. Proliferative breast disease with atypical ductal hyperplasia (ADH) is an indication for chemo- prevention when there is a family history of breast cancer, since there is a 20% risk of developing a malignancy within 15 years. Lobular carcinoma *in situ* (LCIS) is a marker for increased breast cancer risk (25% lifetime risk) as is ductal carcinoma *in situ* (DCIS), which increases a woman's chance of developing a new primary breast cancer to 0.8–1.0% per year. Early neoplastic changes in the breast epithelial cells of these patients may be amenable to modulation, and chemoprevention trials either before definitive surgical excision or after local therapy may prevent in-breast recurrences or new primary cancers. Finally, patients with a history of node-negative invasive lobular or ductal breast cancer, with a good prognosis, and with a low (<15%) risk of recurrence are potential candidates for chemoprevention studies with the goal of preventing a contralateral primary breast cancer as well as an ipsilateral in-breast recurrence.

TAMOXIFEN AND RALOXIFENE

Several large, randomized studies have demonstrated that adjuvant therapy with the non-steroidal anti-estrogen, tamoxifen citrate, reduces the risk of developing a second contralateral primary breast cancer by 30–50%. The National Surgical Adjuvant Breast Project (NSABP) showed a 50% reduction in the incidence of contralateral breast cancer with tamoxifen treatment in node-negative, estrogen receptor-positive patients, as well as a reduction in ipsilateral in-breast recurrences in patients

that were treated with lumpectomy and radiation therapy. However, the estrogenic proliferative effects on the endometrium must be considered with this treatment as it is associated with an approximately 2.3-fold increase in the risk of developing endometrial cancer. Recent reports address this problem and recommend its use only for 5 years to minimize the risk of second malignancy.

The magnitude of a woman's risk of developing breast cancer is being assessed using a risk model which takes into account a woman's age, number of first-degree relatives with breast cancer, nulliparity or age at first live birth, age at menarche, number of breast biopsies, and histologic diagnosis of atypical hyperplasia or LCIS. To have been eligible for the NSABPP-1 Breast Cancer Prevention Trial using tamoxifen versus placebo, a woman must have had a risk profile equivalent to or greater than that of a 60-year-old woman, i.e. a 10% lifetime risk and a 1.7% probability of developing breast cancer in the next 5 years.

A news release from the National Institute of Health (USA) and the National Cancer Institute in April 1998 announced that 'Six years after its inception, the Breast Cancer Prevention Trial (BCPT) shows a 45% reduction in breast cancer incidence among the high-risk participants who took tamoxifen (Nolvadex[®]), a drug used for the past two decades to treat breast cancer. As a consequence, their moral obligation was to notify the 13 388 women who were on placebo of their findings, and told them "...after consulting with your personal physician, you should consider starting tamoxifen" '.

Tamoxifen did increase 'three rare but life-threatening health problems: there were 33 cases of endometrial cancer (cancer of the lining of the uterus) in the tamoxifen group versus 14 cases in the placebo group; there were 17 cases of pulmonary embolism (blood clot in the lung) in the tamoxifen group versus six cases in the placebo group; and there were 30 cases of deep vein thrombosis (blood clots in major veins) in the tamoxifen group versus 19 cases in the placebo group.'

159

Another recent report of chemoprevention indicates that Reloxifene, used for the treatment of osteoporosis in a non-selective estrogen receptor modulator, has estrogen effects on bone and lipids, but estrogen antagonistic effects on breast and uterus, substantially reducing the risk of breast cancer in the postmenopausal woman at risk for the disease, and also may reduce the risk of endometrial cancer.

THE RETINOIDS

The retinoids (vitamin A analogs) are believed to promote mammary differentiation and to decrease proliferation, thus, they too could be considered a chemopreventive agent. Studies are underway to determine their value. The Eastern Cooperative Oncology Group is evaluating tamoxifen versus tamoxifen plus fenretinide (a vitamin A analog) as adjuvant therapy for patients older than 65 years with estrogen receptor-positive, node-positive breast cancer. At the National Tumor Institute in Milan, Italy, DePalo and colleagues have randomized nearly

3000 node-negative patients with breast cancer to receive 200 mg/day of fenretinide versus placebo for 5 years.

OTHER CHEMOPREVENTIVE SUBSTANCES

Other than the anti-estrogens and retinoids, dehydroepiandrosterone, an active adrenocortical steroid, has potential as do the monoterpenes. There are some studies in women already underway for the latter. Asian females with 20–30 times higher consumption of soy beans have much lower breast cancer rates. The isoflavonoids from soy beans are being considered as potential chemopreventive agents.

As for the use of diet to control disease, there have been many papers proposing that coffee may play a role in development of carcinoma and should be avoided. Also, various dietary components including zinc have been suggested to help prevent cancer, but none has definite efficacy.

Bibliography

American Cancer Society 1996 Advisory Committee on Diet, Nutrition, and Cancer Prevention. American Cancer Society guidelines on diet, nutrition, and cancer prevention: reducing the risk of cancer with healthy food choices and physical activity. *CA A Cancer J Clin* 1996; 46: 325–42

Cancer Fax (National Cancer Institute Cancer Data Base). Supportive care/screening/prevention information from *PDQ*, 208/04730, 1996

Doregan W. Follow-up after treatment for breast cancer: how much is too much? *J Surg Oncol* 1995; 59: 211–14

National Institute of Health, National Cancer Institute. *Breast Cancer Prevention Trial Shows Major Benefit, Some Risk; News Release*. Bethesda: NIH, April 1998

Oncology Link@ASCO98. *Raloxifene Reduces Incidence of Breast Cancer by 55–66% and May Reduce Risk of Endometrial Cancer in Postmenopausal Women*. May 1998

O'Shaughnessy JA. Chemoprevention of breast cancer. *J Am Med Assoc* 1996; 275: 1349–53

Index